Central Nervous System Disruptions and Adrenal Fatigue Syndrome

Dr. Michael Lam, M.D., M.P.H.
Dr. Justin Lam, A.B.A.A.H.P., F.M.N.M.

About DrLam.com

DrLam.com is a free public educational website offering cutting edge information on natural medicine. Founded in 2001 by Michael Lam, MD, nutritional medicine expert and board certified anti-aging medicine specialist, the site features the world's most comprehensive scientific, evidenced-based information on Adrenal Fatigue Syndrome.

Dr. Lam's mission is to educate and empower others to take control of their health. You can ask questions about your health concerns online. Because of his willingness to answer specific questions, Dr. Lam has helped legions of individuals learn how to use safe, effective and clinically proven natural protocols for self- healing. This educational service is provided free.

Other resources on the website include:

- Quick 3 minute Adrenal Fatigue Test to assess your adrenal function.

- Our free adrenal fatigue newsletter to keep you up to date on the latest AFS research. Get the latest information presented in easy-to-understand language.

- Hundreds of cutting-edge original special reports and videos by Dr. Lam on everything related to Adrenal Fatigue Syndrome.

- An extensive and archive-rich library of answers to questions previously asked by others that are certain to help you in your recovery from Adrenal Fatigue Syndrome.

- Over 30 conditioned-based health centers with specific clinically proven natural protocols ranging from heart health to cancer.

Dr. Lam offers a worldwide, telephone-based, one-on-one, nutritional coaching service. Personalizing the natural principles discussed in this book, his coaching service has successfully helped countless Adrenal Fatigue Syndrome sufferers recover and reclaim their vitality.

For more information, visit *DrLam.com*
Facebook : www.FaceBook.com/drlamcoaching
Google+: Plus.Google.com/+drlam
Twitter: Twitter.com/drlammd
YouTube.com: www.YouTube.com/user/doctormlam

Contents

Introduction

Other than fatigue and lack of energy, disruptions of the central nervous system (CNS) account for many debilitating symptoms and frequent complaints of Adrenal Fatigue sufferers.

Common symptoms of Adrenal Fatigue Syndrome (AFS) such as low blood pressure can be overcome by increasing hydration; salt craving can be compensated by an increase in salt intake; reactive hypoglycemia can be overcome by an increased frequency of food intake like snacking. No medication is helpful.

Major symptoms indicative of central nervous system (CNS) disruptions include brain fog, anxiety, and severe insomnia. Anxiety during the day with brain fog that reduces mental acuity and productivity; feeling wired at night when it is time to sleep but unable to fall asleep; waking up frequently during the middle of the night with the inability to quickly return to sleep; these are all common occurrences for those with advanced AFS. Few are spared. Sufferers are universally frustrated and in a state of despair. The more advanced the AFS, the higher the risk of developing these CNS disruptions.

Unfortunately, conventional medicine has little to offer other than a sleeping medication, an anti-anxiety agent, and an anti-depressant. While these can be of significant help on a temporary basis, the sad reality is that the vast majority of sufferers develop dependency behavior with time. The end result is a weakened body with worsening fatigue and function as CNS disruption remains unhealed.

This book will present an overview of how the neuroendocrine system is tied to adrenal fatigue and how CNS dysfunction is a central part of this condition. It will also give us a clearer picture of the three key disruptive CNS symptoms of an adrenal fatigue sufferer: brain fog, anxiety, and insomnia.

Chapter 1

Adrenal Fatigue Syndrome: A Neuroendocrine Condition

Stress enters our sphere through a small area of the brain stem called the locus coeruleus (LC) (also spelled locus caeruleus). Discovered in the eighteenth century, this area of the brain stem deals with physiological responses to stress and panic.

As an important homeostatic control center of the body, the LC receives input signals from a variety of sources, including the hypothalamus, amygdala, cerebellum, and prefrontal cortex. Emotional pain and stressors from the outside enter our inner world through these pathways. Once arrived, excitatory signals trigger production and release of norepinephrine from the LC. Norepinephrine has dual functions. In the brain, it acts as a neurotransmitter and keeps us aroused. Norepinephrine released from the LC also increases the sympathetic discharge or inhibs the parasympathetic tone in the peripheral nervous system, exerting its excitatory effects directly on the target organ concerned, such as the heart. As a result, both the force of the heartbeat as well as the heart rate increases. Aside from being the principal production site of brain norepinephrine, the LC is also connected to many other parts of the CNS, including the spinal cord, brain stem, cerebellum, hypothalamus, amygdala, and cerebral cortex.

Collectively, the LC and the areas of the CNS affected by the norepinephrine it produces are described as the locus coeruleus-noradrenergic system, or LC-NA system. Distribution is ubiquitous and consistent with a prominent role for norepinephrine (also called noradrenaline or NA) in a variety of CNS functions and behaviors that include loco motor control, cognition, motivation, and attention.

Activation of the LC-NA system may be responsible for much of the psychological effect we see in Adrenal Fatigue Syndrome, including fear, anxiety, alertness, memory changes, and REM sleep dysregulation. Psychiatric research has documented that the role the LC plays in cognitive function in relation to stress is complex and multimodal. Once activated by stress, the LC responds by increasing norepinephrine secretion, which in turn activates the HPA axis, starting at the hypothalamus. The body then goes on alert and prepares for impending danger.

The hypothalamus is an area of the brain located below the thalamus, just above the brain stem. By its various influences, the hypothalamus plays a key role in controlling hunger, sleep, thirst, circadian cycles, and body temperature. It is the beginning of the hypothalamic-pituitary-adrenal (HPA) hormonal axis. About the size of an almond, it produces and secretes certain neurohormones, one of which we call the corticotropin-releasing hormone (CRH). CRH is released from the hypothalamus when stimulated by norepinephrine from the LC. CRH travels to the pituitary gland and serves as a bridge to link the nervous system to the endocrine system. The neuroendocrine connection is then established.

The pituitary gland is an endocrine gland about the size of a pea and is a protrusion off the bottom of the hypothalamus at the base of the brain. It secretes nine hormones that keep the body in homeostasis. Upon arrival to the anterior pituitary gland, CRH triggers and induces the formation and release of adrenocorticotropic hormone (ACTH). ACTH travels to the adrenal cortex and is responsible for orchestrating the synthesis of a family of steroids including cortisol, the master anti-stress hormone.

The HPA axis works concurrently and alongside the LC-NA system. The HPA axis goes into action when the LC-NA system is activated. While the LC-NA system's effect tends to localize to the CNS, the HPA axis effect is more diffused and affects the entire body, mediated by cortisol and other stress response hormones. This is graphically illustrated as follows:

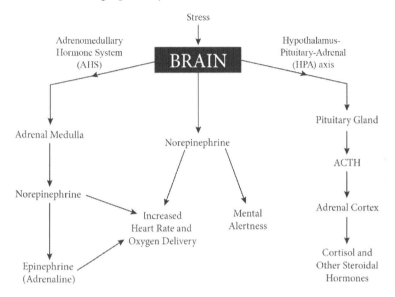

Figure 1. Neuroendocrine Basis of AFS

Therefore, the body has three, well designed anti-stress mechanisms in place to protect us: brain norepinephrine keeps us alert in the CNS, systemic norepinephrine keeps our cardiovascular system ready to take action physically by way of the sympathetic nervous system (SNS), and a family of steroids from the adrenal cortex helps generate energy and reduce inflammation. Activating any or all of these three systems in varying degrees is enough to help us deal with unwelcome stress under most normal circumstances and ensure that our daily living is smooth.

The SNS is part of the autonomic nervous system (ANS), which has five branches. Working together in unison, these five branches regulate the internal housekeeping functions of the body at rest and in emergency. The sympathetic nervous system is responsible for up- and down-regulating many homeostatic mechanisms in living organisms. Fibers from the SNS innervate tissues in almost every organ system, providing at least some regulatory function to things as diverse as urinary output, pupil diameter, and gastrointestinal motility. The other four branches of the ANS are:

- the parasympathetic nervous system (PNS),

- the adrenomedullary hormonal system (AHS),

- the enteric nervous system (ENS), and

- the sympathetic cholinergic system (SCS).

Normal bodily housekeeping functions of daily living are regulated by a perfect balance primarily by the PNS (and its chemical messenger, acetylcholine) and the SNS (and its chemical messenger, norepinephrine). The nervous system is illustrated in the following diagram, Fig. 2:

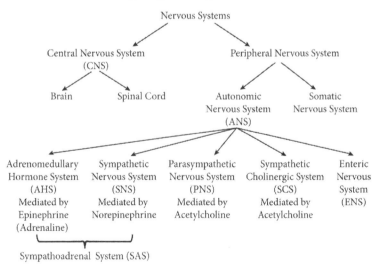

Figure 2. The Nervous Systems

It is absolutely necessary for the SNS to be involved in regulating even small stressors such as standing up or exercise in order for daily living to be seamless. Messages travel through the SNS in a bidirectional flow. Incoming signals carry sensations such as heat, cold, or pain.

Outgoing messages can trigger changes in different parts of the body simultaneously. For example, they can increase peristalsis in the esophagus; piloerection (goose bumps) and perspiration (sweating); widen passages of the bronchi; decrease motility of the large bowel; constrict blood vessels; and raise blood pressure. Thanks to the SNS, LC-NA system, and HPA axis working together each time stressors arrive, individuals in early stages of AFS may experience stress, but seldom notice any significant clinical dysfunction. Working behind the scenes, they help us deal with stress without us knowing about it.

Adrenomedullary Hormone System (AHS) to the Rescue

When stress becomes extreme, the adrenomedullary hormonal system (AHS), also known as the sympathetic adrenergic system, is activated.

What makes the AHS physiologically unique is the way the synaptic pathways are structured.

Synapses occur between pre- and post-ganglionic neurons of the AHS within the adrenal medulla instead of outside the adrenal glands as is the case with the SNS. Because the adrenal medulla develops in tandem with the SNS, it therefore acts as a modified sympathetic ganglion.

The incoming nerve fibers come directly from cell bodies in

the spinal cord. The fibers pass through the para-vertebral ganglia by way of splanchnic nerves without stopping or relaying their signals via cells in the ganglia. This is a direct link highway to the adrenal medulla. The speed of transmission is extraordinarily fast as a result. Furthermore, the post-ganglionic neurons do not leave the medulla. Instead, they directly release a large amount of epinephrine and a proportionally smaller amount of norepinephrine into the bloodstream.

Epinephrine, the most potent catecholamine, serves as an emergency hormone largely responsible for executing the fight-or-flight response, with norepinephrine as a helper. Upon release, epinephrine is carried to the cardiovascular system and other parts of the body. It increases blood glucose levels, increases pulse rate and blood pressure, quiets the gut, stimulates metabolism, and dilates blood vessels in skeletal muscle. At the heart, we see the rate and force of contractions increased. Key organs responsible for getting us out of physical danger, such as the heart, therefore receive excitatory stimuli from norepinephrine directly transmitted through the SNS, as well as both epinephrine and norepinephrine secreted from the adrenal medulla through the AHS. This double protection maximizes our chances of survival in times of danger.

A Gang of Four

From a neuroendocrine perspective, we have four stress response systems well in place within the body from the moment we are born. They are the LC-NA system, HPA axis, SNS, and AHS. In varying degrees, all four systems work constantly around the clock and they balance each other to ensure homeostasis and help us with stress. Multiple feedback loops are in place to help accomplish this mission.

There is a clear and logical pattern of the activation sequence that defines how the body decides which system to activate, to what degree, and under what circumstances. Perceived stress, for example, may be handled differently hormonally than actual stress. Therefore, this gang of four serves an ongoing function to protect and serve our survival needs.

Any one of these systems can be overtaxed and dysregulated. The causes range from toxins, chronic stress, medications, and hereditary factors, just to name a few. Out of these, chronic stress is perhaps the biggest culprit. Overtaxed systems invariably lead to dysregulation and breakdown as a function of time. Symptoms of AFS are merely reflections of such stress response activation, burden, dysregulation, breakdown, compensatory effect, and ultimately, collapse of this regulatory process over time. For example, we see classic signs of hypoglycemia and low blood pressure, both reflective of HPA axis dysregulation, in early Adrenal Exhaustion. Dysregulation of the AHS with epinephrine overload tends to occur later on.

The Neuroendocrine Cascade in AFS

Now that you know the various chemical messengers involved, let's take another look at the stress response from a neuroendocrine perspective, as AFS advances through its various stages. From this cascade, you will see how the body systematically handles different levels of stress with different response systems, all logically. When stress enters the body, the immediate central command of the stress response lies in the brain. Controlled by the LC, mediated through the LC-NA system by the brain neurotransmitter, norepinephrine, the body is aroused and put on alert when stress arrives at its doorstep. This action is immediate and localized to the CNS.

The HPA axis also activates and serves as the messenger chain that ultimately controls the field command center located in the adrenal cortex, where various hormones are produced, including cortisol. These hormones have a diffusive effect throughout the body, increasing energy and glucose, and reducing inflammation. In addition, the SNS is called into action as part of the readiness drill.

The sum of all three systems forms a complex structure and is likely to be involved early on with AFS, though the degree in which each of the systems participates is highly variable and not known. Great overlap is expected, and that signifies a well designed system with multiple control points. Successful deployment of the three systems of stress control in early stages of AFS returns the body to a normal state. Thus, no symptoms are reported by those suffering from Stage 1 and 2 AFS.

If stress is unrelenting, HPA axis signaling is increased. The adrenal cortex workload is put on overdrive. Cortisol output rises. This is Stage 2 of AFS. A persistent high cortisol level has many unintended consequences, the most prominent of which is dyslipidemia and central obesity; both are forerunners of the metabolic syndrome. As Stage 2 progresses, persistent HPA axis over-stimulation and burn out may reach a point where dysregulation is on the horizon.

This point is reached when we enter Stage 3A of Adrenal Exhaustion. Cortisol output is compromised at the adrenal glands by this time. Independently, excessive norepinephrine peripherally may overwhelm the body's other organs, such as the heart and slight cardiac palpitations may surface. The LC-NA system may be over-stimulated as well, if stress is unresolved. With constant brain arousal, a growing sense of being irritable and anxious is common. We also start seeing clinical and subclinical signs of HPA axis dysregulation, including hypoglycemia and low blood pressure. Anxiety, brain fog, and a cognitive toll also increase as the LC-NA system stretches to the limit.

If left unresolved, further deterioration of the HPA axis dysregulation may arise as Stage 3A progresses, triggering other downstream hormonal axes dysregulation as we enter Stage 3B. The dysfunction of one organ system, such as the adrenal gland, can trigger a domino effect, leading to dysfunction of other organ systems. An example of this is the ovarian-adrenal-thyroid (OAT) axis imbalance in women, and the adrenal-thyroid (AT) axis imbalance in men.

The fire now spreads to involve multiple hormonal imbalances, with concurrently low cortisol, low progesterone, and low thyroid. With the HPA dysregulated and the OAT axis imbalanced, the sympathetic nervous system (SNS), already activated before, is now put in overdrive as a compensatory reaction as we enter Stage 3C. Excessive norepinephrine, the key hormone of the SNS, builds up. This can lead to heart palpitations, increased fatigue, and panic attacks. This hormone, normally playing a low key homeostatic regulation function of daily living, now becomes part of the emergency anti-stress team. It is now also responsible for some of the fight-or-flight responses to get the body ready for impending doom and for priming other hormones for action.

If stressors are still not resolved after the above three systems are well deployed, the body, in its final attempt to overcome stress, puts the adrenomedullary hormonal system (AHS) on overdrive. The AHS is already on alert and working behind the scenes as needed from earlier phases. As the body enters late Stage 3C and 3D of Adrenal Exhaustion, the AHS goes on full throttle. A large amount of epinephrine and a smaller amount of norepinephrine are released from the adrenal medulla directly into the blood stream, flooding the body. This ensures that the vital organs, such as the brain and heart, get the necessary blood flow and thus, oxygen, for survival. Other less important systems for survival such as the reproduction and gastric systems are sacrificed temporarily. The AHS is designed to be a temporary emergency stress response of last resort. Long term stimulation without adequate rest may lead to AHS dysfunction, putting the body into a state of further disequilibrium, and at the end, disarray. This frequently appears in sufferers who take metabolic stimulants to keep up their energy when faced with fatigue, not knowing that this strategy can be harmful to the AHS.

If not reversed on a timely basis, the overall anti-stress hormonal supply chain continues to deteriorate. Cortisol and other hormones become grossly dysregulated and severely depleted. This generally occurs in advanced phases of Adrenal Exhaustion. In its last ditch attempt to increase production of hormones, undesirable and destabilizing positive feedback loops may be activated in the process. Crashes are common. If not reversed, the body has no choice but to continue to down-regulate to conserve energy concurrently.

Over time, it draws nearer to failure as it runs out of necessary basic reserve to prime the hormonal pump for normal basic function. To conserve energy, the body admits defeat, surrenders and turns to activating what reserve is left standing as it enters a basic survival mode. This is accomplished by further down-regulation of essentially all bodily functions, the last of which to be sacrificed is the brain. This effectively reduces energy output to a level close to a vegetative state as the final preparation for impending collapse. It comes as no surprise that those with advanced AFS are invariably incapacitated and bedridden.

Who is in Control?

From a neuroendocrinological perspective, it is clear that the body's multiple stress response pathways offer redundancy systems to handle stress the vast majority of the time. It has ensured the survival of our species for quite some time. What is confusing clinically in AFS, is that these pathways can be activated a few at a time, or all at once, and quickly or slowly, as the body sees appropriate for that moment in time. The body is truly in control, despite what appears to be total confusion from a conventional medical logic perspective.

To fully appreciate the body's heroic effort to rescue us from stress, it is important to understand first that our brain is in control of our body through the neuroendocrine system. What one person perceives as stressful may not be for another. Based on the perceived level of stress by the mind, the body automatically activates any or all of the anti-stress mechanisms in place by way of hormones and neurotransmitters.

In order for us to fully grasp the big picture, clinicians and sufferers alike need to take a step back, because it is easy to be confused from a closer or subjective perspective. The picture from afar is crystal clear: a body unable to maintain homeostasis even though it is trying all its ways to recover on its own with the only method it knows — by activating any or all of the built in stress response systems modulated by the neurological and endocrine systems. The more severe the stress, the more other systems, such as the musculoskeletal, psychiatric, cardiac, and immune, are also affected adversely.

The body is a closed system. Severe dysregulation of one system invariably impacts other systems. This is inescapable. Despite this clinical chaos, one can see a controlled collapse that is logical and systematic from the body's point of view. Symptoms are simply the messages or signs the body sends us as warnings of impending danger, thereby alerting us to take appropriate action. Despite a losing battle, if stressors are not removed, the mind continues to be ultimately in charge throughout this ordeal through various neuroendocrinological stress response pathways.

The neuroendocrine basis of AFS is solid and clear. Evidence-based scientific research has proven beyond a doubt that stress can and does kill!

Key Points to Remember:

Stress enters our body through the neuroendocrine system, starting at the brain.

Stress signals the activation of the HPA hormonal axis, leading to the release of cortisol at the adrenal gland.

Dysregulation of any significance will disrupt the body, leading to physiologically unpleasant symptoms, the most prominent of which is fatigue, anxiety, and insomnia.

Chapter 2

Brain Fog and Memory Loss: Metabolite Overload

One of the most common complaints of late stage AFS is deteriorating mental acuity. Cognitive function waxes and wanes, comes and goes. Those in a career that requires a sharp mind, become annoyed and frustrated.

Symptoms include:

- Loss of short-term memory

- Slowdown in common mathematical calculation speed

- Inability to recall names of close friends at times

- Cognitive impairment when under stress

- Increased food sensitivities and intolerance

Brain Fog

The human brain serves as the control center of the neuro-endocrine system.

Subclinical brain dysfunctions can be extremely serious and cause a number of problems in our lives. One of the common issues that people deal with every single day is brain fog. This is a condition where a person cannot think clearly about everyday matters. Though this is a highly prevalent condition, it is rarely recognized or discussed by health practitioners. You won't find brain fog recognized as a bona fide illness in many medical or psychological writings.

The reason is simple—physicians are not taught of its significance in medical school. This under-education leads to tremendous confusion among the public and professionals alike between various memory loss conditions and their differentiation. Brain fog, because of its rather mild presentation, is ignored as a significant clinical condition.

What is Brain Fog? A Clinical Definition

Brain Fog has been described as a feeling of mental confusion where the individual lacks mental clarity. It is as if there is a loss of focus, and a sensation where recall is "so close and yet so far." The term "fog" is used because it feels as if a cloud comes over your thought process, and that reduces your ability to think clearly. This may cause an individual to become excessively forgetful, though long term memory remains intact. It can last anywhere from a few hours to a few days or weeks. Its onset can be gradual or sudden. Usually there is no direct physical trauma to the brain involved. Most people know something is wrong but cannot put their finger on it. Most do not take it seriously and consider it part of life or the aging process. It is considered more of a nuisance among conventional health practitioners.

Brain fog can persist for a long time, lasting months or years. What makes this condition perplexing is that the fogginess can come and go. It can be related to food, menstrual cycle, body temperature, activity level, sleep cycle irregularity, stress, hydration status, exercise, and many other seemingly insignificant events that only become obvious on careful retrospective examination.

Severe brain fog can lead to inferior work performance among those whose careers rely on a high degree of mental acuity. Severe chronic brain fog can ultimately lead to discouragement and depression.

Diagnosis

To date, there are no specific medical tests to diagnose brain fog. Brain scans are normal. Assessment is best made by talking to a knowledgeable doctor about your symptoms. Although symptoms can vary from one person to another, most often, sufferers complain of:

- Lack of mental clarity

- Mild memory loss

- Mental confusion

- Difficulty performing simple tasks like arithmetic or remembering telephone numbers

- Dizziness

Your doctor may have a hard time getting to the bottom of your complaints and the constellation of symptoms can fit many ailments like dementia, Alzheimer's Disease, or mental illness.

There is no objective laboratory test to measure brain fog. It is a subjective clinical determination based on careful history and exclusion of medical illnesses that presents with similar symptoms. Generally, a sufferer has a normal physical examination, but realizes that they do not function as well as they should mentally, but they don't understand why. Most physicians pass it off as an annoyance or natural result of aging with no significant clinical concern.

Your mind may often seem foggy, and your thought processes, slow and cumbersome. Brain fog is not the same as Alzheimer's or dementia. It is also much different than mental retardation, depression and other mental ailments. Since the condition comes on very gradually, sufferers often deal with it as best as they can and do not look for causes and answers to their condition.

What Causes Brain Fog?

In the majority of cases, brain fog is brought on by nutritional, metabolic, hormonal, and biochemical imbalances that stem from a variety of factors.

Toxic metabolic byproducts made up of lipophilic compounds are attracted to the brain and is perhaps the most common culprit for brain fog.

Advanced Adrenal Fatigue Syndrome and Brain Fog

During advanced AFS, the entire body slows down to conserve energy as a survival mechanism. As the liver slows down, the rate of metabolic clearance slows but laboratory tests continue to show normal results. Internal accumulation of unwanted metabolites can travel to the brain, triggering inflammation and a reduced neurological signaling velocity. Information processing is compromised, our thought processes slow and become unclear, and brain fog ensues.

Recovery usually requires a comprehensive program focused on the adrenal glands, a nutritious diet, supplements and lifestyle changes to rebalance the metabolite build-up.

While AFS is frequently associated with brain fog, there are many other possible causative factors that lead to a buildup of unwanted toxic metabolites, as well. We shall examine some of these now:

Yeast Infection

Candida albicans overgrowth produces toxic substances like alcohol and acetaldehyde, which then poisons the nervous system, contributing to brain fog.

An individual may feel like they are confused mentally, although they have consumed no alcohol. Symptoms can drastically worsen from eating too many carbohydrates, processed sugars, starches and fats. Starchy foods and sugars feed yeast organisms, causing them to grow and invade other parts of the body. In extreme cases, the yeast infection can even reach the brain.

During yeast die-off, individuals may experience additional brain fog; this is brought on by a dietary change, fasting, antifungal therapy, or a dramatic lifestyle change. Any change in metabolism can cause yeast to die, therefore releasing a variety of toxins that can overwhelm the body. This condition is usually temporary, but you may experience brain fog during this time.

Hypoglycemia and Brain Fog

Hypoglycemia, also known as low blood sugar, has been associated with brain fog. The glucose level in your brain can become very low, resulting in a brain starved for fuel. Our brain uses a large portion of the calories we consume. Your muscles have the ability to store fuel, but your brain does not. This means it must have a continuous supply. Maintaining a normal blood sugar level in the brain is one of the key survival mechanisms of the body. When the brain's fuel supply varies, all organ system functions are affected.

Symptoms of low blood sugar often occur two to three hours after eating and include:

- Confusion

- Irritability

- Anxiety

- Fatigue

- Dizziness

- Forgetfulness

Laboratory tests of blood sugar may reveal the hypoglycemia, but very few people fall into this category. Instead, most people will show normal blood sugar levels while symptoms of hypoglycemia still are present.

This type of hypoglycemia is called reactive hypoglycemia. It is classically seen in those with advanced AFS.

You can get temporary relief by eating a candy bar or something sweet. The danger of eating sweets each time your blood sugar feels low is that it perpetuates Candida albicans and worsens AFS if the underlying issue is not properly addressed.

Putting the body on a roller-coaster ride of fuel input to prop up energy supply usually triggers more brain fog.

Artificial Sweeteners

Artificial sweeteners such as Nutrasweet® have been shown to cause a number of conditions including brain fog. They can also cause depression, panic attacks, dizziness, fatigue and many other ailments. These substances can be found in thousands of products we all use every day. It is sometimes hidden in products like toothpaste, vitamins, medications, and breath mints. It can also be labeled as aspartame, Equal, Canderel, Spoonful, aspartic acid, phenylalanine, or neotame.

Food Chemicals

For those who are constitutionally sensitive, additives to foods, beverages, and other products can cause problems. These are known as excitotoxins. These substances can be added to drinking water, foods, and common products we all use each day. One of the most common product is MSG (monosodium glutamate). It is responsible for the Chinese Food Syndrome where people develop symptoms of anxiety, dizziness, or brain fog after eating food from Chinese restaurants where MSG use is nearly universal.

There are a number of foods that often cause mild allergic reactions and may lead to brain fog. Not everyone will react to these foods but some people do show low tolerance to foods like spelt, wheat, soy and cow's milk as well as other dairy products.

If you believe you may be suffering from brain fog, then try eliminating them from your diet. More and more individuals are discovering that they are sensitive to gluten-containing foods like oats, rye, barley, wheat, corn, and spelt.

Medications

A number of prescription and over-the-counter drugs contain ingredients that can cause brain fog or mental confusion. Those with sensitive systems should learn to read the labels and know what they are really taking in. Even things like blood pressure medicines, heart medications or drugs for infections and glaucoma can contain irritating substances.

Often, people take several of these drugs at the same time. It is difficult to predict how a combination of drugs may affect a person, but it's never recommended to use alcohol or recreational drugs when taking heart or blood pressure medication.

All types of birth control pills, patchs, and intrauterine devices (IUD) may also cause brain fog for some individuals.

Nutrient Deficiencies

The human brain requires a number of nutrients in order to perform at optimum efficiency. These include proteins, high-quality fats and starches. Our brain also needs minerals and vitamins. Some of the more important ones are magnesium, calcium, zinc, selenium, chromium, thiamine, iodine, L-taurine, choline, L-glutamine, B6, and B12. Omega 3 fatty acids and Vitamin D are also important for good brain health. So when the body is deficient in any of these nutrients, brain fog can be worsened.

B-vitamin deficiencies can result in irritability, confusion, and lethargy. These symptoms mimic those of Alzheimer's Disease. Correcting this is very simple and inexpensive.

Infections

Viral infections affect the brain by excreting toxins into the bloodstream. This results in the depletion of certain nutrients essential to the brain. The viral titer may fall in normal ranges on lab tests, but a sensitive person can feel the difference. Stealth viruses that can directly or indirectly affect the brain include Hepatitis C, Herpes, human papillomavirus, Epstein-Barr, and cytomegalovirus, among others. Infected teeth or gums can also release toxins. Lyme disease as well as H. Pylori infections also frequently trigger brain fog. A chronic, low-grade infection can even arise from a poorly done dental root canal.

Mercury

Most fresh fish worldwide has some level of mercury. Pregnant women and children are usually advised to be cautious about the amount they consume. Those living near coastal regions are particularly vulnerable. Those who consume a diet that includes fish more than twice per week may, over time, build up a toxic level of mercury in their bodies. The Environmental Protection Agency (EPA) recommends that women, children, the elderly, and those with health concerns avoid eating swordfish, shark, tilefish and king mackerel because they traditionally contain higher levels of mercury.

The EPA does recommend limiting your consumption of these fishes to two meals per week. They also advise checking local authorities about the mercury levels in fish caught in local lakes and ponds before eating any freshly caught fish.

Another common source of overlooked mercury is dental fillings. A biological dentist is needed for proper removal in these cases if the body is ready. Overzealous removal of mercury fillings can trigger brain fog as mercury released from the oral cavity travels to the central nervous system.

Mercury is a neurotoxin. Excessive build up can lead to numerous neurological symptoms including memory loss, tingling, and brain fog, among others. Fortunately, mercury levels in the body can easily be determined by a blood test.

Copper

Those with excessive levels of copper in their bloodstream may experience mood swings, confusion, or feelings of disorientation. Their thought process may be muddled or race in many directions. Women may notice that the condition worsens just before and during their menstrual period. This time of the month is usually marked by higher cellular activity which increases copper levels in the blood.

Regular use of birth control pills or patches can worsen this problem. A copper imbalance can affect other areas as well, including your thyroid. Copper imbalances are normally difficult to diagnose. A doctor can administer special blood and urine tests to tell if you have high levels of copper.

Hair tissue mineral analysis can reveal high copper levels as well. If you've been experiencing consistent migraine headaches for years with no explainable cause, this can indicate high levels of copper.

Although not absolute, indicators that can infer the presence of high copper toxicity include high calcium, potassium, mercury, and zinc levels in the blood or hair tissue.

Copper imbalances can occur for many reasons. Some of these include vegetarian or semi-vegetarian diets, stress, zinc deficiency, using birth control pills, fatigue, or copper IUDs. Some areas also experience copper contamination in drinking water or food, due to pollution.

Most vegetarian diets are low in zinc and high in copper. These diets are often low in other essential nutrients that are important for proper brain function. These include carnitine, taurine, B12, essential fatty acids, and others. Those who suspect they may have brain fog should avoid a vegetarian diet and try to eat at least one portion of animal product each day, and see if their brain fog resolves.

Other Toxic Metals

Brain fog can also be brought on by toxicity with other metals, such as aluminum, lead, cadmium or others. Aluminum is found in antacids, antiperspirants, soda-cans, and many cosmetics.

Commonly recommended metal detoxification modalities include chelation, cleanses, enemas, flushes, saunas, hot soaks, massages, and others. Medications like EDTA and DMPS are also used. IV Chelation is the most common and recognized way to reduce heavy metal in the body. Not everyone can tolerate or do well with chelation. It can cause a detoxification reaction among those who are weak or sensitive, such as those in advanced stages of AFS or Chronic Fatigue Syndrome. Aggressive metal detoxification is a common clinical mistake in those with advance AFS and can trigger adrenal crashes.

Petrochemicals

Even without overload of heavy metals such as mercury, most people are exposed to some level of toxic petrochemicals these days. They occur everywhere, from the interior of your auto, such as the plastic dashboard and seat cushions, to common plastic items found around the home such as plastic shampoo containers and other plastic bottles. Other less obvious items include products used on your lawn, inks, paints, and even insecticides used in growing our fruits and vegetables. Most city water supplies have various levels of toxic chemicals and these are usually monitored by your city water treatment facility. In larger cities, even the air is polluted, as well.

Many manufacturing plants also utilize processes that include chemicals and other harmful substances in their manufacturing process. These can include cleaners and lubricants.

Over a number of years, these chemicals and their toxic metabolites can build up in the body's bloodstream and major organs, and become a dangerous issue. This is especially true when a person doesn't eat right, doesn't get enough exercise, or uses nicotine products. These things weaken the body and make it difficult for the internal bodily functions to operate correctly. The bottom line is that the body stops filtering the harmful substances out on a regular basis and they begin to build up internally. Because most metabolites are fat derived, they tend to be lipophilic. They like to stay in the brain which is also lipophilic because like-compounds attract each other. An excess of these lipophilic compounds in the brain, unable to be cleared out by the circulatory system, is a major contributing factor to brain fog.

Bowel Toxicity

Improperly digested foods can ferment or rot in the intestines. This, in turn, generates a number of powerful toxins. These substances will slowly poison the liver and other major organs critical in the detoxification process, resulting in an increase in toxic metabolite by products traveling to the brain and causing a diminished capacity to think clearly.

Food consumed by the body needs to be processed and excreted out on a timely basis. This transit time is usually under eight hours, but can take up to 20 hours or more if one is constipated. Once it goes past 20 hours, the foods in your gastrointestinal system will start to rot, releasing toxic substances into your bloodstream. When the process of assimilation and metabolization is slowed due to AFS, these toxic metabolites tend to build up internally.

Alarming signs of this include consistent constipation or slow bowel transit time. Enemas may be needed in severe cases to help a bowel movement. Slow bowel passage can be alleviated by using products that add fiber to the diet, enhancing of liver function, drinking lots of water, and alkalizing the body. Diet should also be altered to include foods that are high in fiber and low in sugar and fat. Magnesium can be helpful as well.

Gluten Intolerance

Gluten is a protein found in many grains, including wheat, rye and barley. Foods that contain gluten can cause unusual reactions in the brains of those with gluten sensitivity. Any type of food allergy can disrupt the sensitive balance of hormones and chemicals in our brains. The results can range from depression to schizophrenia.

Those sensitive to gluten may suffer from malabsorption and irritable bowel syndrome (IBS), which leads to low levels of essential nutrients in the body. In these cases, your body attacks the gluten as if it were an invader, and this damages the finger-like projections known as villi which are part of the intestines. These villi absorb nutrients as your food passes through the small intestine.

Our brains require wholesome foods and water along with a variety of nutrients to be completely healthy. Some of the required vitamins and minerals include calcium, B12 and B6, zinc, selenium, iodine, and vitamin D.

These nutrients can be found in a wide range of foods, but they may not be digested properly if you are gluten sensitive. This makes it important to find out if you are gluten-sensitive and eliminate these foods from your diet. You will quickly notice an improvement in your mood, learning skills, digestion, and other areas.

Electromagnetic Field (EMF) Sensitivity

Everyone is different and some people are more susceptible to electrical and electromagnetic fields. Though they are quite harmless to some, they adversely affect others. They can disrupt sleep patterns and cause a decline in overall performance at work or school. This type of brain fog originates from sitting in front of a computer screen for long periods or the excessive use of cell phones. Those who live near cell phone towers, electric plants, or radio towers can also be affected. These objects emit invisible electromagnetic rays (waves) of energy that can cause certain sensitive people to feel upset or distressed.

It's a good idea to turn off all televisions, computers, radios and other electrical devices well before and while sleeping. If possible keep electronic devices at least 10 feet away from your brain while sleeping. Unplug all electronic devices when not in use.

Psychogenic Causes

In some cases, brain fog can be caused by mental and emotional conflict or serious trauma. For instance, if you've been in a severe family conflict or accident where you or someone you love was injured, then you might continue to experience a condition similar to posttraumatic stress disorder (PTSD) for some months afterwards.

You feel disconnected, like you can't think clearly about ordinary things. In cases like this, the individual uses brain fog as a way to deny reality. This can occur when your life isn't going well. Perhaps you are going through a divorce or bankruptcy and your stress level is very high each day. Our bodies and brains find ways to deal with these adverse situations.

If the situation doesn't improve, it may warrant speaking to a licensed therapist or psychologist. Sometimes all we need is a little help to get through particularly harsh circumstances.

Other Causes of Brain Fog

Misalignment of the spine can cause headaches and backaches. These can be hereditary or caused by trauma such as an accident. When the cranial or cervical nerves are pinched or out of alignment, this may not only cause pain, but it can also contribute to brain fog. Cranial-sacral therapy and chiropractic manipulation may be helpful in these cases.

Reduced oxygen to the brain is another culprit and this can simply be due to not breathing deeply and filling the lungs with fresh air each day. Too many of us sit in stuffy offices and never get outside to take deep breaths and enjoy the sunshine (which is physically beneficial as well). Reduced oxygenation can also be caused by clogged arteries or low blood pressure. Certain diseases such as chronic bronchitis, COPD, asthma, or emphysema also impair adequate breathing. Always make sure your upper airways are in good condition as the nasal passage is connected to and part of the overall respiratory system.

There are a few other illnesses and ailments that can, in rare cases, cause brain fog. These include but are not limited to brain tumors, meningitis, epilepsy, or encephalitis. Some vision problems may be a contributing factor, along with dyslexia and autism. The mental confusion that goes along with dyslexia, autism and ADHD often results in brain fog. Fortunately, these are quite rare.

Electrolyte imbalances due to excessive sweating during exercise or physical labor will sometimes cause temporary brain fog. When the sodium level in the body is low, thinking is affected. It's always a good idea to stay hydrated especially during the summer months with salt replenishment as needed.

Brain Fog and Adrenal Fatigue Syndrome

Brain Fog first and foremost is a symptom and not a disease in the context of AFS. Living in the modern world with much toxicity and pollution requires a body with excellent metabolic pathways to reduce toxic load. This is a 24/7 job, with much of the burden falling on the liver. When the adrenals are weak, the body's way to restore health is to conserve as much energy as possible once the self-repair mechanism has been exhausted.

The process of self preservation during survival triggers a series of metabolic slowdowns in order to save enough needed energy for essential daily function.

When the body's metabolic pathways slow, liver congestion and extra cellular matrix pollution increases. The body can be overloaded with unwanted metabolites unable to be removed on a timely basis. Some of these toxic metabolite are carried to the brain by the body's circulation and therefore impair clarity of thought.

Most metabolic byproducts are steroidal compounds at their molecular level. They are lipophilic, a term used when a compound is attracted to fat. They are therefore attracted to the most fat-loving parts of our body, the brain and central nervous system. These unwelcomed visitors then trigger inflammation as the body tries to get rid of them. Swelling and slowed neuron conductivity are natural consequences at the subclinical level. Unfortunately, there is no gross pathology detected and brain scans are deemed normal. Yet the brain appears to be "bogged down" with reduced mental acuity and reduced speed of thinking.

The more advanced the AFS, the more a person is at risk for brain fog.

Correcting Brain Fog

Because brain fog is a sign of underlying dysfunction, the most important correction step must start with a physician who is alert to all the possible symptoms and pays close attention to your history. Brain fog usually has a strong metabolic component in the case of AFS, and usually spontaneously resolve once adrenal health improves.

Laboratory tests are generally not very helpful and can in fact be confusing to interpret. Marginal abnormalities are common. Proper clinical correlation is an absolute must. It is easy to get carried away trying to treat the laboratory numbers rather than the person. It is important to remember that not every single laboratory abnormality needs to be corrected, and an aggressive correctional protocol can actually generate unwanted side effects which could make the overall condition worse. Those who are in advanced stages of AFS are particularly vulnerable due to the prevalence of paradoxical reactions that can surface.

Aggressive detoxification therapies commonly deployed for brain fog include enemas, cleanses, flushes, infrared sauna, acupuncture, reflexology, deep tissue massage, nutritional supplementation, herbs, chelation, and intensive chiropractic therapy. Fasting is also very popular. These can be considered for those in good health with constitutionally strong bodies when properly conducted under supervision. Those who are weak or sensitive can get worse with any of these programs quickly. Self-navigation with these short term approaches is not recommended. A longer term comprehensive program done professionally, focusing on metabolic nutrition is usually needed for permanent results.

In a context of advanced AFS, short term approaches to fixing brain fog often will backfire unless the adrenals are well healed. Proper timing is key. Those in advanced stages of AFS will do much better by focusing on the root cause first and making sure that a nutritional reserve is built prior to attempting any aggressive detoxification procedure to avoid triggering adrenal crashes. This is a much safer and more effective long term strategy.

We do see many cases of brain fog that spontaneously resolve once adrenal dysfunction is repaired properly and naturally without the use of stimulants. Patience is required. Most are pleasantly surprised on how fast the body can respond if the proper adrenal recovery program is instituted.

Key Points to Remember:

Brain fog is a common, but subtle and unrecognized condition of cognitive impairment. It is characterized by a nonspecific feeling of confusion, loss of short term memory, and difficulty performing mental calculations.

A variety of factors including nutritional, hormonal and metabolic imbalances can contribute to the dysregulation of the neuroendocrine system and hamper cognitive function, giving rise to brain fog.

Sufferers in advanced stages of AFS often complain of brain fog. Often, building the body's strength with nutritional reserves and addressing adrenal dysfunction will resolve symptoms of brain fog over time.

Chapter 3

Wired and Tired: Neurotransmitter Dysregulation

Without a doubt, most advanced Adrenal Fatigue Syndrome (AFS) sufferers report daily struggles with their emotional and cognitive health. The role neurotransmitters play in this cannot be underestimated. In addition to fatigue, many report a sense of anxiety throughout the day, while feeling tired at the same time, often due to the lack of proper rest at night. This sense of being "wired and tired" is an accumulation of multiple physiological factors, many of them mediated by neurotransmitters.

Here are some common signs that your neurotransmitter levels may be in imbalanced or dysfunctional:

- Inability to fall asleep

- Frequent awakenings in the middle of the night and inability to return to sleep

- Adrenaline rushes

- Waking up unrefreshed

- Being easily excited and easily depressed

- Having the blues

- Loss of appetite

- Weight loss for no apparent reason

- Gastric bloating

- Jittery hands

- Ineffectiveness of sleep aids such as melatonin
- Reduced effectiveness of strong sleep medications
- Heart palpitation at rest or when sleeping
- Crashing after intense exercise
- Prolonged recovery time required after sex
- Reduced libido
- Feeling better with coffee or drugs such as adderall
- Feeling calm after Adrenal Breathing Exercises
- Feeling excited after taking a hot bath
- Nightmares or vivid dreams
- Inability to do work that requires mental focus

Neurotransmitter Balance and Adrenal Fatigue Syndrome

Neurotransmitters (NTs) are chemicals in the brain that act as messengers, transmitting signals between the neurons, allowing communication to take place with the multitude of organ systems functioning within the body. These are potent neurochemicals that regulate nearly every function in the body including physical and cognitive performance, weight, the perception of and response to pain, sleep patterns, and our general emotional and mental state of being.

Scientific research reveals that malfunctions in neurotransmission, such as an imbalance, deficiency, or disruption, are very common these days and are the root cause of many common health conditions. When our NTs are not working in optimum balance, our mind and body cannot communicate clearly and effectively. It is estimated that about 80 percent of people have some form of NT imbalance. Fortunately, only a small number are clinically symptomatic and debilitating.

Brain function is affected whenever there is dysfunction or poor functioning of NTs, or malfunctioning hormonal axes that are the ultimate conduit upon which NTs exert their effect, such as the hormonal hypothalamic-pituitary-adrenal axis (HPA). In this chapter we will examine both defects in a setting of AFS.

How our Nerves Communicate With Each Other

Before we can fully comprehend the effect NT problems can have on us, we first need to understand why they are critical for communication. We can compare our nervous system to the electrical system in our homes. Nerve cells communicate with each other via tiny circuits called neural pathways. What's different is that our nerve cells don't touch each other; they come very close but there is a gap between them called a synaptic cleft. The neuron sending the message is the presynaptic cell or axon, and the neuron receiving the message is the postsynaptic cell, or dendrite.

The direction of communication is one-way, and to send the message across the synapse from the presynaptic cell to the postsynaptic cell, chemicals called neurotransmitters are used. For example, a typical synaptic transmission using the NT serotonin would involve the following events. A presynaptic cell produces serotonin from tryptophan (an amino acid), and accumulates the serotonin into small vesicles, which are in the terminals at the end of the axon. When your brain sends a signal (an action potential) it goes down the presynaptic cell and arrives at the end terminals. Upon arrival, serotonin is released and fills the synaptic cleft, crosses and binds with its serotonin receptors located on the surface of the postsynaptic cell on the other side. When there is adequate serotonin binding to its receptors, a certain minimum threshold level is attained, and the signal (action potential) will arrive in the cell and continue to be propagated by moving on to the next cell. The goal is for the signal to reach its intended target and generate a response.

To avoid having the nerve in a constant state of being on, the excess serotonin molecules in the synaptic cleft are eliminated by monoamine oxidase (MAO) enzymes plus a process called catechol-O-methyl transferase (COMT). Some of the remaining serotonin does return to the presynaptic cell in a process of absorption called reuptake. As the serotonin level reduces, the nerve signal is turned off and the system resets to baseline. The communication system is now ready to receive another signal or action potential. Some classes of antidepressants block the serotonin reuptake process, leading to increased serotonin. They are called SSRIs or selective serotonin reuptake inhibitors. They include drugs such as Lexapro, Prozac, Paxil, and Zoloft.

Neurotransmitters 101

The body's main neurotransmitters are:

- Dopamine (DA), acting as precursor to norepinephrine and epinephrine

- Norepinephrine (NE), the workhorse NT for the sympathetic nervous system

- Epinephrine (E), also known as adrenaline, the workhorse NT for the sympatho-medullary nervous system

- Acetylcholine (ACh), the NT for the parasympathetic nervous system

- Serotonin (5-HT), the body's feel good NT

We now study each of these in more detail, starting with a group called catecholamines. Catecholamines are a grouping of NTs, which are often referred to as the stress hormones. They are all derived from tyrosine, an amino acid. These NTs have the ability to act faster than cortisol, a hormone that responds to stress. The key catecholamines are dopamine, norepinephrine, and epinephrine.

Dopamine is a vital NT as well as a precursor to norepinephrine. Dopamine released in the brain acts as a natural reward for pleasurable experiences such as having sex or dining on a delicious meal. It can also be released in response to neutral stimuli resulting in pleasure becoming associated with those stimuli.

When dopamine is released in excess amounts in the brain, the effects can be anxiety, hyperactivity, and paranoia.

When dopamine levels are low, the effects can be addiction, cravings, compulsive behavior, depression, and inability to concentrate or focus.

Norepinephrine (NE) is an important NT that helps to regulate attention and arousal, and plays a part in the fight-or-flight response. It acts both as a NT and a hormone. In the brain, it functions as an excitatory NT, putting the body in a state of mental alertness. It is produced and acts in the brain to prepare the individual to deal with a perceived threat. It also travels outside the brain. Once outside, it acts as a hormone and plays an important role in increasing heart rate and blood pressure, dilating pupils, dilating air passages in lungs, and narrowing blood vessels. It is the main controller that facilitates the actions required for day-to-day stress control that we take for granted, such as standing up quickly from a reclining position without feeling dizzy.

If someone is living under ongoing stressful conditions, a long-term excess of norepinephrine in the brain can result. Such is the case of AFS, especially in the moderate to advanced stages. Chronic excess of norepinephrine is called sympathetic overtone. It can cause cellular and tissue inflammation, raise blood pressure, cause symptoms of hyperthyroidism, and trigger panic attacks.

On the other side of the spectrum, if there is a deficiency of norepinephrine over a long period it may cause behavioral problems, secondary hypothyroidism, immunological imbalances, and impair cognitive functioning.

Epinephrine (E) is a key NT in the physiological fight-or-flight reaction in response to an immediate threat when survival is perceived to be at risk. It is the chemical daughter of norepinephrine. Their actions are similar, but epinephrine is far more potent. This hormone is secreted in the adrenal glands under the direction of the HPA axis and produces a rapid rise in blood pressure, and heart rate, and stimulates the release of glucose in the liver. This is the hormone of last resort for the body when it is in imminent danger. The more danger the body is perceived to be in, the more epinephrine will be released. Those who are in very advanced stages of AFS are constantly flooded with epinephrine internally. Symptoms include heart palpitations, dizziness on standing, and panic attacks.

Acetylcholine (ACh) is a major NT for the parasympathetic nervous system (PNS) and helps the body carry out the day-to-day housekeeping functions of rest-and-digest or feed-and-breed activities that occur when the body is at rest, especially after eating. These include urination, sexual arousal, bowel movements, and digestion.

Serotonin is a monoamine NT synthesized in specific neurons in the brain, the central nervous system, and in enterochromaffin cells located in the gastrointestinal tract. It is also called the feel good NT. Inside the brain, the raphe nuclei is the center for serotonin production. Throughout the entire central nervous system, serotonin has a vital role in modulating a number of different areas:

- Anger

- Aggression

- Appetite

- Body temperature

- Erection and ejaculation

- Mood

- Sexuality

- Sleep

- Stimulation of vomiting

Serotonin is also a precursor to melatonin. Once they have completed their task, a reuptake or reabsorption of these hormones takes place. Serotonin is effective in making us calm and basically helping us feel good. It helps the mind to relax so that we can easily fall asleep and stay soundly asleep.

Serotonin and melatonin are produced in the body from tryptophan, an amino acid. A person who doesn't have any serotonin cannot produce abundant amounts of melatonin. The ability to convert from one type to another depends on a variety of nutritional cofactors and coenzymes.

For a person to feel well, the overall serotonin level cannot be too high or too low. Chronic excess of serotonin over a long period of time may result in:

- Behavioral problems

- Cardiovascular problems

- Hormonal and immunological imbalances

A long-term depletion or deficiency in serotonin can cause:

- Depression

- Gastrointestinal problems

- Hormonal imbalances

- Imbalances in the immune system

- Inflammation

- Insomnia due to low melatonin

- Onset of various medical conditions

Neurotransmitter Precursors

The compounds utilized in the manufacturing of NTs are called precursors. Anything affecting the precursors will in turn affect the resulting NTs and influence how the nervous system functions in the end. If there is a deficiency in a specific precursor, then that can cause a bottleneck in or delay the creation of a particular NT and affect its ultimate functionality. It is also true that if there is an excess of a certain precursor that can cause the resulting NT to have excessively high levels.

- Precursors of dopamine (DA), norepinephrine (NE) and epinephrine (E): DOPA, phenylalanine, tyrosine

- Precursors of serotonin (5-HT): 5-HTP, tryptophan

- Precursors of acetylcholine (ACh): phosphatidylcholine, acetyl group amino acids such as N-acetyl-L-cysteine (NAC) or acetyl-L-carnitine (ACL)

Neuromodulators

There are a number of different neuroactive substances

working to promote the proper functioning of the NT. The following are some and their contributions:

- Ascorbic acid (vitamin C)—an anti-oxidant
- Histamine—mediates allergic and pain reactions, also acts as a potent vasodilator
- L-Aspartic acid—an excitatory amino acid
- L-Glutamic acid—an excitatory amino acid
- L-Lysine—works to prevent extracellular matrix destruction

NT precursors and modulators serve important functions. They are generally less potent and thus available as over-the-counter nutritional supplements. Their gentle character allows them to be used in cases where medications such as NT repletion tools are not indicated or well tolerated. They are also less addictive because they tend to be weaker in action.

Inhibitory vs. Excitatory Neurotransmitters

NTs generally fall into two groups when classified by their actions:

Inhibitory NTs—Serotonin, glycine, and GABA fall into this category. When we have plenty of these in our system we feel good. These NTs also assist with our sleep and contribute to our self-esteem. When these become depleted in our system we can become angry, depressed and suffer from insomnia.

Excitatory NTs—These NTs keep us focused, alert, motivated, and help our memory. They include catecholamines (dopamine, epinephrine, and norepinephrine), and glutamate. A low level of dopamine causes impaired short-term memory, a low sex drive, difficulty with numbers and general fatigue. A shortage of norepinephrine will bring on depression, a lack of motivation and ambition, and an increased likelihood of becoming dependent on caffeine and other stimulants. If we have too much norepinephrine we can arouse panic and have difficulty sleeping. Many recreational street drugs work by stimulating this pathway.

For the body to be in optimum health, these opposing camps of NTs need to be perfectly balanced.

L-Glutamate (glutamic acid) is the most vital excitatory NT functioning in the brain and performs a significant role in brain chemistry. It is released by a variety of neurons and acts to stimulate other neurons. The more glutamate, the higher the levels of excitation. If the excitatory NTs reach excessively high levels, a state of excitotoxicity exists. This is when the neuronal activation has reached such a high level that the stimulated firing of neurons has become neurologically damaging.

On the other end of the spectrum, molecules such as GABA and taurine are part of the inhibitory NTs. GABA is derived from glutamine and synthesized when the active form of vitamin B6 (P5P) is present. Inhibitory NTs inhibit or prevent the firing of neurons. It plays a critical role in the regulation of neuronal excitability throughout the entire nervous system so that the body does not operate on a continuous high or state of excitement. They reduce anxiety and promote calmness.

Symptoms of Neurotransmitter Imbalance or Deficiency

There are currently over sixty different mental and physical illnesses associated with a deficiency or imbalance in NTs, including:

- Addiction in any form, including sex, sugar, gambling, drugs, alcohol, caffeine, smoking (nicotine), carbohydrate addiction and/or binge eating

- Advanced stages of AFS
- Fibromyalgia
- General malaise
- Irritable bowel syndrome
- Memory impairment (forgetfulness)
- Obsessive-compulsive disorder (OCD)
- Parkinson's disease
- Tourette's syndrome

In particular, neuroscience research has uncovered strong associations between low levels of serotonin and/or norepinephrine with the following mental conditions:

- ADD/ADHD
- Anorexia
- Anxiety
- Bulimia
- Chronic pain
- Depression or mood disorders
- Fibromyalgia
- Insomnia or sleep disorders
- Migraines
- Obesity

- Panic attacks

- Premenstrual tension

- Restless legs syndrome

- Bipolar disorder

- Cognitive disorders

- Depression

Causes of NT Deficiency, Imbalance or Malfunction

There are a number of different reasons why people have imbalanced levels of NTs in their system:

- Diet. The depletion of NTs may be caused by poor dietary choices. NTs are made from amino acids that in turn are derived from protein, vitamins and minerals in diets and supplements. If there is a deficiency of these vital ingredients, there will be a deficiency in the level of NTs in the system. Practicing vegans or vegetarians on a low protein diet are more prone to NT deficiencies.

- Unsuitable nutrients. They can also be problematic. Caffeine and sugar top the list of foods most harmful for NTs. They affect the brain in much the same way as hard drugs. Junk food and foods made from white flour also cause damage to NTs.

- Toxic Consumables. Alcohol, nicotine, mind-altering drugs, ephedra and ephedrine are some medications that can lower the effective action of NTs. Phentermine (used in the fen-phen diet years ago) actually causes long-term damage to the receptors for serotonin. This means that you need to have even higher levels of serotonin in your system to get the benefits of the NT. This was why many people on the fen-phen diet gained their weight back and more when they went off the diet.

People with NT deficiencies or imbalances experience a variety of symptoms and often use alcohol and/or drugs to deal with their discomfort as a form of self-medication. This might provide some initial relief, but the problem is exacerbated because this only causes further damage and depletes their natural production of NTs even further. In addition, prolonged use carries the risk of dependency.

- Sensory Overload. The brain is constantly bombarded with sensory overload from noise, radio waves, rapid visual stimulation from computer monitors, TVs, movies, fluorescent lights, etc. When all this electronic light flickers faster than the eye is able to detect, the brain is required to work harder to modulate all the incoming stimulation in order to remain focused on the task at hand. More NTs need to be produced which can ultimately lead to exhaustion and thus depletion.

- Environmental Toxins. Everyone is exposed to toxins in the environment and even inside our homes, every single day. We use cleaning products, laundry soap and fabric softeners, air fresheners, perfume and cologne, nail polish, and other personal care products. We are exposed to pesticides and herbicides in our garden and construction products if our home is undergoing a remodeling. Our indoor and outdoor carpeting contains chemicals and so does our clothing. All of these things contain toxic chemicals that can seriously affect our NTs. These toxins can directly affect the receptors and even inhibit our natural production of NTs.

- Genes. There are certain individuals who are born without the essential enzymes for synthesizing NTs. These people naturally have deficiencies or dysfunctional NTs. Serotonin transporter genetic defects, for example, have been associated with child maltreatment.

- Bowel Dysfunction. Since the majority of NTs are in the gastrointestinal tract, any sort of GI dysfunction could be a major cause of NT depletion. They include:

  - Candida—yeast overgrowth

  - Congestive bowel toxicity

  - Inflammatory bowel syndrome (IBS)

  - Leaky gut syndrome—increased permeability in the intestines

- External and Internal Environmental Factors. NT balance can be altered by many external factors, such as rapid change in barometric pressure. Many have reported onset of depression after a visit to a high altitude environment. Internal factors can include any of the following:

  - Head cold or sinus congestion

  - Hepatobiliary dysfunction (liver congestion)

  - Ingesting foods that one is sensitive or allergic to

  - Polluted extracellular matrix

  - Rapid changes in hormone levels

- Rapid changes in blood sugar

- Chronic Stress. Stress has the effect of raising blood pressure, insulin levels and the activity of free radicals in the body. All of this damages the neurons. Chronic stress is especially damaging to our overall NT production, regulation, and control. Our body operates on a system of checks and balances, which keeps everything in alignment. When we are under stress, such as someone with advanced AFS, excitatory NTs such as catecholamine levels may increase. This is especially prevalent in advanced stages of AFS where the body is flooded in a sea of norepinephrine and epinephrine (adrenaline). As a compensatory response, the body will release more inhibitory NTs like GABA and serotonin to calm the body down.

If we are under chronic stress and are releasing these NTs on a regular basis, the body becomes desensitized to them, production and release is downregulated and levels are reduced. This leads to a relative catecholamine dominance, an excitatory state, leading to anxiety, insomnia, and depression.

Diagnosing NT Imbalance

It is fairly easy to determine the levels of most NTs in the body by testing a sample of urine. However, interpreting the results is not easy and often can be very confusing because the clinical correlations are not clear or definitive. For example, levels of NTs in urine vary rapidly in reaction to both stress chemistry and diet-related changes that affect the pH.

Although cerebrospinal fluid (CSF) testing provides the actual NT levels available in the brain, it is used primarily in research laboratories. Blood platelet levels of serotonin and the catecholamines have long been known to be reliable NT indicators, as their testing results track closely to CSF testing results. Urine and plasma test results do not correlate well with CSF. Serotonin and catecholamines are stable in blood platelets but not in blood plasma where the levels are extremely reactive to stress.

Some NTs, like acetylcholine, cannot be accurately measured in blood and urine since choline doesn't easily cross the blood/brain barrier. Therefore, it is possible for acetylcholine to exist in high levels in body tissue, but not be at the same levels in the brain where it is needed most.

Urinary GABA levels are particularly hard to decipher. Testing of many stressed-out patients usually show GABA in excessive amounts, yet most of these patients show clinical benefit from GABA supplementation.

Other valid reasons why particular NTs may be outside their reference range would include:

- When NTs are used they are destroyed and this process takes much longer than the production process, which results in higher levels of the NTs when measured.

- Due to a fungal or yeast infection, a NT can be transformed into a false form but still measured in laboratory tests.

- Both viral and bacterial infections can destroy NTs, lowering the real value.

- Other NTs or certain neurochemicals can suppress a NT, lowering the real value.

- If the supply of oxygen is decreased to some parts of the brain, the NTs will be affected.

Clearly, sensitivity and specificity of NT testing via urine has much room to improve and it is a science still in progress. Therefore, clinical correlation is key to making the most sense out of laboratory studies, as they could be misleading and confusing on their own.

Restoring NT Imbalance

NT deficiencies can be repleted with amino acids, and diet and lifestyle changes. NT excess can be helped by lifestyle modifications as well as compounds that calm NT release. It all comes down to balancing so that the excitatory NTs are in balance with the inhibitory NTs. Bias in any direction is not desirable. Most NT imbalances reflect underlying pathology. Comprehensive long term strategies of NT rebalance need to also correct the underlying root causes.

To correct specific NT imbalances, what is needed is to first identify the defective pathway. Clinicians experienced in NT physiology find that a detailed history usually provides the best information to commence NT repletion when depletion is suspected. Expansive testing may not be needed provided the patient is closely tracked and monitored by an experienced clinician. NT imbalance usually presents in a set of clinical behaviors with generally recognizable patterns. Experienced clinicians will be able to ascertain this.

If sufficiently based on history, clinical rebalancing trials should start by stimulating one or more of the specific conversion pathways that may not be working properly, and then observe the results. The key is to first to be able to recognize the symptoms pattern when presented. For example:

- Serotonin deficiency symptoms include: depression, worry, anxiety, obsessive thoughts, PMS, heat intolerance, fibromyalgia, fatigue, and panic attacks.

- Melatonin deficiency symptoms include: sleep onset insomnia, disturbed sleep, and night owl behavior.

- Dopamine / norepinephrine / epinephrine deficiency symptoms include: depression, fatigue, caffeine cravings, lack of concentration, attention deficit.

- GABA deficiency symptoms include: being uptight, feeling burned out, muscle soreness, feeling overwhelmed.

To replete what is deficient, nutritional supplements such as amino acids, vitamins and minerals are used to form a nutritional cocktail that can be taken orally provided the body can tolerate it. Adaptogenic herbs such as maca, rhodiola, and ashwagandha as well as glandulars can play a supporting role when indicated. Other supportive modalities or therapies include electromagnetic therapies that work on the body's qi (energy) as well as brainwave entrainment technologies, bio-feedback, mitochondrial fortification, liver decongestion, extracellular matrix cleanse, and various detoxification techniques designed to enhance the body's self-healing and rebalancing ability when they are deployed at the right time.

The difficulty one encounters with NT repletion in advanced AFS is titrating the right dosage to match the body's weakened state. Inappropriate dosage is a common cause of adrenal crashes and setbacks. This is a common clinical mistake.

Along with nutritional repletion, here are eight lifestyle changes that can help NT imbalance:

Lifestyle NT Balancing Tools

1. Gradually Decreasing or Avoiding Antidepressants: Most popular antidepressants are classified as SSRIs, which refers to the selective serotonin reuptake inhibitors mentioned earlier. SSRIs cause short-term flooding of serotonin in the brain. Along with this, there is a quick degradation of serotonin while it remains in the synaptic cleft. The result is that more and more serotonin is eventually needed since the receptors for serotonin become desensitized to the constant fluctuation of NTs. However, the body begins producing less and less natural serotonin since it has started to depend on the medication which provides an external source of serotonin. When the brain does release its own serotonin, it is degraded very quickly since the enzymes left in the synaptic cleft are now trained to quickly break down any serotonin.

Many taking antidepressants will need constant dosage increases. As this occurs, the body depletes a fair amount of the receptors in the brain for serotonin. Furthermore, the receptors for serotonin in your colon, kidneys and liver can be damaged. This affects the sensitive balance between your gut and your brain, which regulates appetite, creating a vicious cycle.

Those who are already on SSRIs should not stop abruptly as that can cause unpleasant withdrawal symptoms.

2. Minimize Coffee Intake and Other Stimulants: It has been shown that small amounts of caffeine can enhance mental performance and guard against the onset of Alzheimer's, so it need not be avoided entirely except for people who are at risk for or suffering from AFS. Caffeine can affect the brain in a similar manner as antidepressants or other central nervous system stimulants such as ephedra or ephedrine. They can overwhelm

the brain with excitation which can create a resistance and/or long term damage to NT receptors.

If you really must drink coffee, you should try to limit yourself to an eight to ten ounce cup of black coffee a day. One week every two months you should switch to decaf coffee. People who rely on coffee, tea, energy drinks or even soda change their brain chemistry and certain physical characteristics over time. Caffeine is fat-soluble and easily crosses the blood-brain barrier, so as you drink more and more coffee, the caffeine causes your brain cells to produce more NT receptors for adenosine. What adenosine does is bring about a feeling of being tired. The structure of caffeine resembles that of adenosine very closely, which means that caffeine can readily fit into the receptors in your brain cells for adenosine. With caffeine always plugging the receptors for adenosine, adenosine can't bind to its own receptors any longer and bring about the feeling of tiredness. The problem is that the body will respond by creating more adenosine receptors which means you will need to increase your intake of caffeine in order to not feel tired, building tolerance over time.

You can avoid this and kick your caffeine habit by hitting your reset button on your adenosine receptors. You only need to survive seven to twelve days without caffeine, and this is why the recommendation is to take a break from coffee and other stimulants for a week every few months.

Other metabolically stimulating compounds include but are not limited to: thyroid replacement hormones, DHEA, pregnenolone, testosterone, pituitary glandulars, adrenal extracts, green tea, maca, rhodiola, ginseng, zinc, copper, selenium, iodine and kelp. These should all be carefully scrutinized based on need.

3. Keep a Nutritious Diet: The building blocks of many NTs are amino acids, B vitamins, and various minerals. If you are deficient in any of these critical components, you can be left

without the building blocks you need for healthy and balanced NTs.

Some of the best sources of high quality amino acids are almonds and almond butter, free-range eggs, grass-fed beef, quinoa, raw organic dairy products, spirulina or chlorella, and wild salmon. Healthy people with problems sleeping or with motivational issues linked to issues with their NTs can often, but not always, benefit from using essential amino acids.

For the nervous system to function properly to synthesize and circulate the NTs being produced from the precursors and amino acids, you should be taking in adequate amounts of B complex vitamins—vitamin B6, B12, and folate—from food sources. These are extremely important in the metabolic processes in nerves. Good sources of vitamin B6 can be found in bell peppers, spinach, and turnip greens. Good sources of folate can be found in asparagus, beets, broccoli, calf's liver, lentils, mustard greens, parsley, romaine lettuce, and spinach. Good sources of vitamin B12 are found in calf's liver and snapper. External supplementation is acceptable for those who are healthy if you are concerned about whether you have enough. Because of their excitatory nature, those who are weak or sensitive need to be very careful not to take too much.

4. Avoid Exposures to Environmental Toxins: Environmental toxins can detrimentally affect the production of NTs and cause you to be overly sensitive to NTs, which can lead to brain fog, fuzzy thinking and brain damage. These toxins can be found in the mycotoxins existing in moldy coffee, fragrances in perfumes and colognes, and/or the air freshener sprayed around the home or hung in the car. In addition to damaging NTs, toxins also place excessive stress on the liver, causing congestion. The extracellular matrix becomes polluted as well. Neither is conducive to optimal health.

To avoid toxins, here are a few tips:

- Buy organic fruits and vegetables to avoid the pesticides. Otherwise wash all fruits and vegetables in a solution of vinegar and water.

- Use only natural cleaning products, such as vinegar, baking soda, lemon juice, etc.

- Use only natural products for personal care, avoiding dyes, fragrances, etc.

- Use filters in your home for air and water.

Because our body has an intrinsic system of toxin removal, you will start to gradually feel better as you take the steps to avoid further insult. Once you adapt to these changes, you'll find yourself being very sensitive to your NTs being under attack. For example, strolling through the perfume section of a department store has an immediate effect on you. Avoiding toxins should therefore be a lifelong endeavor.

5. Avoid Excess Sensory Stimulation: In the 21st century, we are constantly bombarded by rapid visual images, sounds, auditory input from televisions, computer games, movies, and electronic monitors that flicker so fast the eyes can hardly detect what's in front of them. There are radio and EMF waves, LED and fluorescent lighting, and a hectic lifestyle to contend with. All of this stimulation requires the brain to modulate the constant sensory bombardment at a level that would have never been imagined by our ancestors.

The brain must find a way to calm itself down and use its delicate supply of serotonin and GABA, the calming, inhibitory NTs. All of this overstimulation impacts NTs and their receptors significantly, so think about the following activities you may be doing:

- Listening to loud music while working out

- Getting involved in exciting, fast-moving or violent video games or movies before going to bed
- Playing computer games for several consecutive hours
- Staring at a computer monitor for most of your workday
- Listening to background music
- Constantly using artificial, fluorescent lighting in your home or workplace

6. Repair and Protect Your Gut: Your gut is second only to your brain in influencing bodily functions. Your gut actively uses over thirty different NTs as it contains your enteric nervous system. The truth is that 95 percent of your body's supply of serotonin exists in your gut. Consider that in the distance from your esophagus to your anus there are approximately one hundred million neurons. This is more than in your spinal cord or your entire peripheral nervous system.

The lining of your gut produces NTs; and the bacteria in your gut, numbering in the billions, are also creating NTs. What this means is that if the lining of your gut is damaged in any way, or the flora is not in balance, then you are at risk for an imbalance in your NTs or even deficiencies. The reason why so many people suffer from irritable bowel syndrome at one time or another is an overabundance of serotonin in their gut, which means they have an imbalance in the NTs there. This explains why taking antidepressants can cause such serious gut problems. Maintaining healthy flora with probiotics is therefore an important part of a comprehensive NT balancing program as long as it does not trigger constipation.

7. Smother Nerves in Healthy Fats: Your NTs are only as good as their ability to help in the transmission of signals. This is largely the function of the myelin sheath. Myelin sheaths wrap around your nerves, and in order to have a healthy nervous system you should take in certain nutrients which will

help support the production of these protective myelin sheaths. Not to mention good myelin sheath production supports your nervous system in general. A good quantity of omega-3 fatty acids, specifically docosahexaenoic acid (DHA) can be helpful. DHA is extremely important in forming the structure of myelin sheaths and in the prevention of the breakdown and degradation of nerve cells. Excellent sources of omega-3 fatty acids can be found in flax seeds, kale, collard greens, walnuts, and winter squash. However, the quantity of DHA that the body absorbs from plants, nuts and seeds is really quite low.

There are better sources of omega-3 fatty acids and DHA that are more readily available, which include cloves, cod, halibut, grass-fed beef, salmon, shrimp, sardines, and tuna. For vegetarians or vegans, algae-based DHA supplements are recommended, such as the ones from marine phytoplankton. Other sources of food that support the formation and health of neuronal membranes and myelin sheaths include almonds, avocados, macadamia nuts, olive oil and pecans. This is because of their high concentrations of oleic acids

8. Mindfulness, Yoga and Breathing: Mindfulness is the act of being more aware and conscious of the present moment, non-judgmentally. Or, in other words, making a conscious choice to be aware and experience the present moment to the fullest without judgment in all your activities, without dwelling in the past or the future. The frequent use of mindfulness is one of the most effective methods for reducing stress, managing chronic pain, alleviating depression and anxiety, coping with life, overcoming addictions. To top it off, it is a great avenue for spiritual development, self-actualization, and creativity. Mindfulness helps boost and balance our feel-good NTs like dopamine, serotonin and endorphins, and at the same time reduces excessive norepinephrine, the NT associated with chronic stress.

The Adrenal Breathing Exercise is an excellent, clinically proven tool that brings mindfulness to calm the overactive autonomic nervous system when under stress. NTs responsible for breathing rhythm include GABA, glutamine, and glycine. Proper breathing not only rebalances NTs, but also prevents overexcitation of the sympathetic nervous system that leads to excessive release of norepinephrine and epinephrine. Adrenal Breathing Exercise is specific in accomplishing both and is an invaluable tool. It should be an integral part of the NT balancing program and its power should not be underestimated.

Research has shown that practicing yoga may elevate brain GABA levels, the brain's primary inhibitory NT. This suggests that the practice of yoga should be explored as a possible treatment for depression and anxiety disorders associated with low GABA levels. Yoga has shown promise in improving symptoms associated with depression, anxiety and epilepsy. The Adrenal Yoga Exercise series is designed specifically to calm the autonomic nervous system and rebalance NTs without excitation of the sympathetic nervous system.

Neurotransmitter Repletion Prescription Medications

The two main classes of NT repletion medications designed to overcome depression and anxieties are SSRIs and SNRIs. SSRIs include drugs such as Citalopram (Celexa), Escitalopram (Lexapro), Fluoxetine (Prozac), Paroxetine (Paxil and Pexeva), and Sertraline (Zoloft). SNRIs include desvenlafaxine (Pristiq), duloxetine (Cymbalta), and venlafaxine (Effexor and Effexor XR).

SSRIs work by inhibiting the reabsorption of serotonin. By causing the body to feel good, they ease symptoms of moderate to severe depression and anxiety disorders. SNRIs work by inhibiting the reabsorption of not one but two important brain chemicals: serotonin and norepinephrine. These drugs are sometimes called dual reuptake inhibitors, or dual-acting antidepressants, and tend to be a bit stronger than SSRIs. Because SNRIs affect two NTs, they may be an effective form of treatment for those who have failed to respond to single-acting antidepressants, such as SSRIs. Some research suggests that patients with severe depression may respond better to an SNRI.

Possible side effects for both SSRIs and SNRIs include nausea, muscle weakness, tremor, heart palpitation, increased blood pressure and heart rate, headaches, dry mouth, fatigue, excessive sweating, constipation, and fluid retention. Women who are nursing or pregnant should avoid taking SNRIs, as they are passed into breast milk. Certain SSRIs may be better options for pregnant or nursing mothers. People with liver problems or high blood pressure will need liver function monitoring periodically via blood tests. Those on aspirin, non-steroidal anti-inflammatory drugs (NSAIDs) such as ibuprofen, and blood-thinning medications such as warfarin (Coumadin) should use SNRIs with caution as SNRIs may inhibit blood clotting, thus increasing the risk of severe bleeding from a cut or scrape.

One of the major problems associated with both SSRIs and SNRIs over time is dependency as well as exacerbating NT depletion, the very problem it is supposed to solve.

In time, more and more medication is required causing greater and greater depletion leading to a vicious cycle of progressively more medication needed with less and less effectiveness. Typically, there is a short honeymoon with lessening symptoms of depression within the first few weeks. Six to nine months later, however, a rude awakening begins. The patient literally wakes up to returned depression. The patient tries to quit the SSRI, such as Zoloft, and finds that they feel worse than ever. The SSRI never solved the underlying problem of NT deficiency but simply temporarily increased the level of NT by blocking its metabolism at the synapses. As more SSRI enters the system with daily intake, the MAO system increases breakdown of serotonin without the additional nutritional intake of serotonin precursors required for replenishment. The overall intrasynaptic levels of NT gradually decline; and when they fall below the threshold needed to keep the patient disease free, the depression returns with vengeance.

This problem can be resolved by prescribing the proper amino acids and nutrients—the building blocks of NTs—and the benefits of the medications will resume within one to two weeks. Sadly, this is seldom the path taken by conventional medicine. Instead a larger dose or more potent medication is prescribed, again masking the underlying root problem of NT depletion. Over time, sufferers become overmedicated and sedated, but depression continues.

Those who are currently on SSRIs and SNRIs should not abruptly stop their treatment to avoid withdrawal symptoms that can be very hard to bear. Take a step back and look at the big picture. A comprehensive plan is needed to replenish deficiency and rebalance NTs to prevent depression from worsening. Underlying chronic problems commonly associated with NT imbalance, such as chronic fatigue, infection, or AFS, should be addressed so the root cause is dealt with properly. Natural compounds can be administered, but titrated to match the body's state of function at each step along the way. Medications can be tapered off slowly as the body returns to optimal function and root problems resolve. Timing is key, and premature cessation can bring on withdrawal and other negative side effects. Remember that an NT imbalance is more often than not secondary to some other underlying disease, which is why most

NT imbalances self correct once the underlying condition is resolved.

Natural Neurotransmitter Repletion Supplementation

NT repletion can be achieved with the use of natural compounds for those low on specific NTs. This can be accomplished by way of nutritional supplements, in particular, amino acids that are the foundation precursor or modulators of NTs. Athletes trying to achieve peak performance heading into an intense workout or competition requiring extreme focus sometimes take five to ten grams of amino acid powder to fortify themselves. Amino acid supplementation, however, can cause over-stimulation and trigger crashes if the body is weak. They can lead to insomnia and panic attacks. Amino acid supplements include 5-HTP, DLPA, DPA, GABA, glutamine, L-theanine, tryptophan, or tyrosine.

There are many ways to achieve NT repletion, as the following examples will show:

- To increase serotonin—use 5-HTP or tryptophan. Approximately 10 percent to 20 percent of the low-serotonin individuals do poorly on 5-HTP (but do well on L-tryptophan). Some individuals are very sensitive and need to be started on and maintain very low doses of 5-HTP and/or L-tyrosine.

- To increase GABA — use glutamine or L-theanine.

- To increase dopamine and norepinephrine — use tyrosine.

- To increase endorphins — use DLPA or DPA.

Amino acid repletion is usually taken in conjunction with

a variety of other vitamins and minerals because they work together and need one another to support good brain function. For example, pyridoxal-5-phosphate is needed for the conversion of tryptophan to serotonin.

Repletion therapy must be carried out carefully and no one should take matters completely into their own hands without the proper guidance. Most failures occur at inexperienced hands. For example, if you take 5-HTP and no other supplement(s), or if you take improperly balanced 5-HTP, you can easily deplete the dopamine in your system. If you take L-DOPA alone, or improperly balanced L-DOPA, you can easily deplete the serotonin in your system; L-tryptophan, sulfur-based amino acids, and tyrosine do this as well.

Natural Neurotransmitter Repletion Toolbox

1. B Vitamins: For those that need assistance in the methylation processes of melatonin and the catecholamines, the amino acid S-Adenosylmethionine (SAMe) can help; or you can try methionine and vitamin B12. An active form of vitamin B12 can be found in Methyl-B12, so it can be helpful as well.

Active forms of B vitamins are more potent since they are more useable than non-active forms. The active forms don't need to be converted into the form that the body actually uses. They can be utilized by the body as they are, or with fewer steps. This is a benefit for those who are strong and healthy; however, they may be too excitatory for those with weak adrenals. B vitamins therefore have to be carefully chosen to match the body's condition to be successful.

NT repletion supplements can be found in the following B vitamins:

- Active vitamin B6 — pyridoxal-5'-phosphate (P5P)

- Active vitamin B9 — 5-methyltetrahydrofolate (5-MTHF)

- Active vitamin B2 — flavin mononucleotide (FMN)
- Active vitamin B3 — nicotinamide adenine dinucleotide (NAD or NADH)
- Active vitamin B5 — pantothenic acid or pantethine

Alert: Too much vitamin B can trigger crashes. Those who are weak and sensitive have to be extra careful. Side effects include anxiety, heart palpitations, and insomnia.

2. 5-HTTP: Because serotonin does not cross the blood-brain barrier, it cannot pass into its specified pathways in the central nervous system when taken orally. However, the amino acid tryptophan, along with its metabolite 5-HTP or 5-hydroxytryptophan, which serotonin is derived from, does have the ability to cross the blood-brain barrier.

It is not usually advised that tryptophan be taken as a supplement, but 5-HTP is recommended widely as an effective serotonergic agent and is largely safe when taken in small doses. It is helpful to take 5-HTP before bedtime in order to help you relax before going to sleep. It can give you enough serotonin so that the melatonin you need can be produced. For some, it is also helpful to take small doses of 5-HTP throughout the day to help in the production of serotonin and to keep you relaxed.

Recommended dosage: When starting out with 5-HTP it is very important to begin with a very low dose and gradually work your way up. The dosage between individuals can vary from 50 to 200 mg per dose, depending on the person's needs and what they can safely tolerate.

Alert: High dosages of 5-HTP (e.g., 200 mg or higher) may cause nausea and stomach cramps. This is why some prefer to take slow-release 5-HTP supplements at bedtime. These symptoms may only occur at certain points in the day, e.g. at bedtime and not during the day, during the night or in the early hours of the morning if more is taken then. When taken in extremely high doses, 5-HTP can cause serotonin toxicity or serotonin syndrome, and this can be fatal.

3. Melatonin: Melatonin is a hormone made from serotonin. 5-HTP is a precursor to serotonin and thus can increase melatonin levels. In order to produce melatonin and the required coenzymes and cofactors, the body requires a certain amount of serotonin as a primer. A certain level of serotonin in the body is needed to relax enough to go to sleep. When melatonin is produced internally after sleep has initiated, it helps the body stay asleep. A deficient production of melatonin can result in anxiety and mood disorders, lowered basal body temperature, insomnia, elevated estrogen/progesterone ratio, and immune suppression associated with cancer. Excess melatonin is associated with seasonal affective disorder (SAD), lowered estrogen/progesterone ratio, low thyroid and adrenal function, and hypotension.

Melatonin is widely used as a sleep aid. The sleep promoting effects of melatonin are most apparent only when a person's melatonin levels are low. In other words, taking melatonin is not like taking a sleeping pill or even 5-HTP. It will only produce a sedative effect when melatonin levels are already low. By enhancing sleep quality, melatonin enhances NT stability and balance.

Alert: When taking melatonin, you have to be very careful regarding the dosage. Some people are able to absorb and assimilate melatonin quite easily and thus only need a fraction of a milligram. Other people need as much as 50 mg to get the desired effect. In other words, the effect is not a linear response. Some trial and error is required in the hands of an experienced clinician. Those who experience a hangover in the morning with melatonin should take it two hours before sleep rather than at bedtime.

4. GABA, Glutamate, Glutamine: The NTs in the brain doing most of the work are glutamate (also called glutamic acid)

and GABA. Over 50 percent of the synapses in the brain release glutamate, while 30 to 40 percent release GABA. GABA is inhibitory and calming. Glutamate is excitatory and stimulatory. In healthy individuals, GABA and glutamate will be in balance in the brain in their absolute concentrations as well as their relative ratios. Problems arise if the ratio is imbalanced. For example, if GABA production is reduced, a higher glutamate to GABA ratio in the brain will increase, leading to a sense of being wired. A GABA deficiency over time is linked to the following excitatory or stimulatory effects:

• Anxiety

• Behavioral problems

• Imbalance in the immune system

• Insomnia

• Memory problems

If GABA is deficient in the body, it can be repleted using a supplemental form of GABA. Each of us may have different absolute amounts of GABA in the brain that is normal for us. There are no accepted medical tests to determine if we have too much or too little GABA activity. Excessive use of street drugs, alcohol, and prescription drugs are associated with low GABA activity and thus a state of excitation. Caffeine, in particular, inhibits the release of GABA and allows the increase of excitatory NTs.

GABA, glutamine and glutamate are intimately involved in a cycle that ultimately determines the level of each in the body. Neurons are not able to perform new synthesis of the NTs glutamate and GABA from glucose. The glutamate-GABA-glutamine cycle is a metabolic pathway that describes the release of glutamate or GABA from neurons, which are then taken up into astrocytes (star-shaped glial cells). In return, astrocytes release glutamine to be taken up into neurons for use as a precursor to the synthesis of glutamate or GABA. This cycle therefore determines whether more GABA or more glutamate is produced.

Think of glutamic acid, glutamine and GABA as three members of a close-knit family with three very different personalities. Glutamic acid is a non-essential amino acid (the body can manufacture it when everything is working properly) that is also an excitatory NT. Its cousin GABA has the opposite personality—it calms our nerves and relaxes us. Glutamine is the source of both of them—the body can make either glutamic acid or GABA from glutamine, depending on what is needed. Glutamine, therefore, is the gatekeeper chemical that determines the amount of GABA and glutamate levels to be produced to keep them in balance.

If you are in a state of anxiety caused by sympathetic overtone (as commonly seen in advanced AFS) or a severe inflammatory state, production from glutamine will shift to favor GABA to calm the body. This will in turn lower your glutamate level and further help calm you down. Unfortunately, this pathway can be disrupted when the inflammatory state causes dysregulation of the cycle itself, leading to excess production of glutamate levels instead.

This is why it is very hard to predict the overall net effect of glutamine and it is not unusual for a wide variety of outcomes when taken by seemingly homogeneous populations. The negative effects occur most frequently in a body with chronic weakness, such as one with AFS. This may explain why some people do well with GABA supplements, but others can have paradoxical reactions. Similarly, glutamine is also used to support GI health, but it may increase glutamate and cause anxiety as a side effect.

Generally speaking, if you keep the total amount of glutamate in your body under control, you can prevent excitation responses. For example, excessive glutamate such as in Chinese food prepared with the flavoring enhancer monosodium glutamate (MSG) can cause nervousness, headaches, numbness, facial pressure, and anxiety in what is known as the Chinese restaurant syndrome.

Excessive GABA can result in a number of detrimental effects including:

- Breathing problems
- Immune system imbalance
- Impairment in muscular movement
- Memory problems
- Onset of any number of medical conditions

Recommended dosage: Take 100 to 1000 mg in divided doses. GABA is commonly elevated in sufferers with advanced AFS, but it is not clear why. Supplementing with GABA may not seem wise in these conditions, but many have clinically reported benefits, especially for daytime anxiety control. Taking L-theanine is a lot more helpful in this situation and probably safer. It is weaker, as it needs to be converted into GABA and serotonin. It is not recommended that GABA be taken in high doses (500 mg or more) at bedtime as it can cause an alert state and possibly stimulate the production of other NTs that may prevent falling asleep.

5. L-Theanine: L-theanine is another amino acid and a precursor to serotonin. It also helps in the production of GABA and dopamine. Theanine is related to another non-essential amino acid, glutamine. It is considered to be psychoactive since it has the ability to penetrate the blood-brain barrier.

L-Theanine can be taken as an alternative to GABA or L-glutamine to support a calming of the brain. L-theanine is converted to several useful calming and mood-elevating substances in the brain, including GABA. Therefore, one can use theanine as an indirect pathway to bypass the blood brain barrier issue with respect to GABA.

Because L-theanine is known for helping to relieve stress and provide relaxation it is used in some sleep remedies in conjunction with low dose 5-HTP, GABA, melatonin, and calming herbs like passion flower and valerian root.

Recommended dosage: Take 200 to 400 mg once or twice daily. Those with advanced AFS need to be on alert for paradoxical reactions. Stop supplementation if this occurs.

6. Taurine: Taurine is an amino acid that calms the nervous system by facilitating the production of the NT GABA. By helping to raise GABA levels, taurine allows the body to manage anxiety so that your thoughts don't go spiraling out of control and you don't experience the associated cortisol and epinephrine spikes seen in AFS.

Take taurine for better sleep, but make sure you are getting a magnesium supplement that your body can absorb as well. Together, these nutrients abolish stress, calm the nervous system, and help you sleep better. You'll also have an overall improved mood. People who are deficient in either magnesium or taurine are at greater risk for depression and poor motivation.

Magnesium is a well known supplement to calm the nervous system as well as counter fatigue. Taurine raises GABA levels, similarly calming the nervous system and lowering anxiety and stress hormones that hinder rest.

Recommended dosage: A dose in the 500 to 2000 mg has shown efficacy; the upper limit for toxicity is much higher than this and high doses are well tolerated. The upper limit for which one can be relatively assured no side effects will occur over a lifetime has been suggested to be at 3 grams a day. Taurine is a natural diuretic and may cause excessive urination and drop in blood pressure in high amounts.

7. Glycine: Glycine is one of the most common amino acids found within human proteins. It is particularly important clinically in supporting healthy digestive and central nervous systems and combating chronic fatigue. Within the central nervous system, glycine works together with taurine and GABA as an inhibitory NT. It interferes with the hyperexcitability of the CNS neurons by regulating chloride and potassium balance. It has been shown to be beneficial for disorders such as hyperactivity, anxiety, obsessive-compulsive disorder, schizophrenia, bipolar disorder, and epilepsy. Due to its neuro-inhibitory effect, glycine calms the brain and is thus helpful in treating depression and insomnia as well. Glycine also helps in supplying glucose to the body to help alleviate fatigue.

Recommended dosage: Take 1 to 3 grams for anxiety or sleep. Up to 100 grams is needed for schizophrenia.

8. L-DOPA / Tyrosine: L-DOPA has the capability of penetrating the blood-brain barrier and is the precursor of dopamine. Dopamine is involved in the production of norepinephrine, which is converted into epinephrine. Supplementing with L-DOPA can increase the levels of dopamine in the system, but it won't necessarily increase the levels of norepinephrine over the levels of epinephrine. Many factors are involved in balancing the equilibrium in the nervous system so it isn't that straightforward.

Instead of supplementing with L-DOPA, you can supplement with the amino acid tyrosine, which is a precursor of L-DOPA. Tyrosine is contained in many different proteins but it is not as effective since it must go through an additional step in order to produce L-DOPA. Tyrosine supplements may be considered for someone with below normal tyrosine reference ranges and if there are no clinical contraindications.

Recommended dosage: Take 500 to 5000 mg daily in divided doses. Up to 20 grams has been used by researchers to improve cognitive function.

Alert: Overuse of tyrosine can push the body into an over-excitatory state and trigger an adrenal crash, panic attack, and heart palpitations. Don't take L-tyrosine if you have problems with chronic headaches or bellyaches because the supplement might trigger these conditions. If you have problems with hyperthyroidism, such as with Graves' disease, avoid tyrosine.

9. Neuromodulators and Precursors: The following are commonly used:

- Estrogen directly influences brain function through estrogen receptors located on neurons in multiple areas of the brain. At neuronal synapses, estrogen increases the concentration of NTs such as serotonin, dopamine, and norepinephrine. It affects their release, reuptake, and enzymatic inactivation. It also increases the number of receptors for these NTs.

- Phenylalanine (PHE) is a precursor to catecholamines such as dopamine, norepinephrine and epinephrine. If an amino acid analysis shows that levels of phenylalanine are low, then supplementing with it or eating foods rich in phenylalanine may be of help. Foods rich in PHE are meat, poultry, fish, dairy, soybeans, seeds and nuts. Aspartame, an artificial sweetener is also rich in phenylalanine but this is not advised. In general, PHE is seldom recommended because there are superior alternatives.

- Phosphatidylcholine (Lecithin), N-acetyl-L-cysteine (NAC), and acetyl-L-carnitine are all precursors to acetylcholine, the NT of the parasympathetic nervous system.

- Phosphatidyserine (PS) is derived from soy lecithin, a component of cell membranes. PS is helpful in repairing damaged cell membranes as well as repairing the cortisol receptors located in the hypothalamus. When cortisol levels are too high it is believed this elevation damages the receptors, which impairs the hypothalamus' ability to detect when levels of cortisol are too high and to correct the problem. The stronger the phospholipid layer of the cell, the more efficiently the NTs can be transported. PS can be used successfully to help calm elevated cortisol levels at night and induce sleep. Nonetheless, for reasons that are not well understood paradoxical responses are common.

As simple as it may seem, most self-navigating natural NT repletion programs fail, just as most medications that attempt repletion of NTs also fail over time. In particular, those who are under stress are at risk of failure. Sufferers of AFS are highly vulnerable, especially in advanced stages when their HPA hormonal axis is deranged. It is clear that a body under stress will negatively impact the effectiveness of any NT balancing program and in particular, SSRIs. A comprehensive NT balancing program must take this into account to be successful. Let us study why.

How the HPA Axis Affects our Neurotransmitters

The hypothalamic-pituitary-adrenal (HPA) hormonal axis connects sensory signals (such as smell) received from the outside world into NT signals in the brain. The signals then travel to various organs and trigger the release of over fifty hormones that help the body deal with daily living and stress. Remember that stress can be physical or emotional. Moreover, perceived stress is a more powerful trigger of the HPA axis than actual stress. With chronic stress, the HPA axis is put into overdrive, and over time, the adrenal glands become overburdened. If the situation is not relieved, the adrenal glands begin to tire and exhaust.

Advanced AFS is the end result of the body's neuroendocrine response to chronic stress. In early stages of AFS, output of the anti-stress hormone cortisol from the adrenal cortex rises as the adrenal glands are put in overdrive because of the HPA axis. In advanced stages of AFS, cortisol depletion sets in as the HPA axis becomes dysregulated and the adrenal glands reach exhaustion. This is when adrenal epinephrine and brain NT norepinephrine output take center stage as the body enters the flight-or-fight alarm response.

Neurotransmitter Balance and Adrenal Fatigue Syndrome

HPA axis dysregulation in advanced AFS is associated closely with improper NT regulation. For one to function properly, the other must be in balance and synchronization. Without proper balance, the overall condition can easily worsen.

For example:

- Because it increases serotonin, 5-HTP is widely used to make you feel better. Your body maintains a balance of serotonin and cortisol production. Your adrenal glands—the hormone glands responsible for cortisol production—contain receptors that sense the levels of serotonin in your bloodstream. Upon exposure to serotonin, your adrenal glands release cortisol into your bloodstream. As a result, taking 5-HTP—and increasing your body's serotonin levels—also affects cortisol and increases your body's cortisol levels. This can be detrimental to someone who is suffering from early stages of AFS where cortisol output is already higher than normal. Further increase in cortisol can lead to a catabolic state.

- Increases in glutamine will lead to increased glutamate, the excitatory NT. This effect is undesirable as most suffering from advanced AFS are already in an excitatory state from excessive circulation of norepinephrine and epinephrine. Further excitation can increase fatigue and trigger adrenal crashes. Furthermore, glutamine also suppresses cortisol release. At a time when cortisol production in the adrenals are depleted and more is needed, glutamine use is contrary to the body's need for increased cortisol output as part of AFS recovery from advanced stages.

- Many people have negative outcomes when they take 5-HTP and glutamine as well as L-theanine. These are supposed to raise GABA, an inhibitory NT and reduce anxiety commonly experienced by those suffering with advanced AFS. However, these three compounds often cause paradoxical reactions instead. They can trigger adrenal crashes and further overstimulation of the excitatory pathways instead of inhibiting it for reasons not yet understood. This negative chain reaction can make a whole range of symptoms much worse. The reverse can also happen. Taking in more GABA when laboratory levels already show high GABA levels may produce clinically positive results of relaxation for reasons not known.

NT research and understanding is still very much in its infancy. There is much we do not know. What is clear is that NTs are very much interconnected with each other. While we have a solid understanding on the individual physiology of each NT, overall clinical outcomes remain hard to project with accuracy. This is especially true in the advanced AFS setting or for those at risk due to concurrent chronic conditions in which the body is already on edge and alarmed. The slightest change in NT levels can upset the tenuous internal NT balance. Any additional disruption to the already fragile internal homeostasis, such as receptor disorders or extracellular matrix congestion, can lead to exaggerated or paradoxical responses. Severe anxiety and fatigue can be triggered as the risk of an adrenal crash increases.

An example of this is with selective serotonin reuptake inhibitors (SSRIs) used as antidepressant medications, which are very helpful in treating panic attacks. SSRIs cause serotonin levels to rise. Unfortunately, this is not an effective way of treating stress over time because tolerance usually develops; and even with more antidepressants the body becomes desensitized to the added availability of serotonin during neurotransmission, and depression and fatigue persists. This negative scenario is frequently seen in people who are put on antidepressants by their private physician while AFS is overlooked, resulting in a worsening of their depression.

NT Balance Strategy When HPA Axis Imbalance and AFS are Present

When HPA axis dysregulation, NT imbalance and advanced AFS are all present at the same time and the autonomic nervous system is in high gear, the clinical picture becomes very convoluted and complex. For example, overemphasis on NT repletion can trigger excitotoxicity and cause adrenal crashes. Too little NT repletion can retard the overall AFS recovery. Too much adrenal support can trigger NT excitation, and too little adrenal support will lead to increased NT repletion dependency. Regular NT pathways are disrupted in a body that is fragile and sensitive.

A carefully planned and balanced approach starts with taking an in-depth history, with focus placed on both NT repletion and helping the body heal from AFS concurrently. The more advanced the AFS, the more focus and priority should be placed on healing the AFS first.

Amino acids and herbal remedies can be detrimental if the adrenals are not stabilized first or if the liver is congested and the extracellular matrix polluted. If you want to decrease your levels of norepinephrine while at the same time increasing serotonin levels, certain supplements would not be advised. For example, people often try to treat depression by supplementing with St. John's Wort; but if they have extremely high levels of norepinephrine, this can further increase their norepinephrine levels via their association with the HPA axis which can be put in overdrive while supplementing.

Sometimes people use melatonin to help them sleep. Melatonin production begins by turning on sympathetic nerve pathways in the brain that secrete the NT norepinephrine, which in turn stimulates cells in the pineal gland to produce melatonin. This may not be problematic for some, but for those with advanced AFS where the body is already flooded in a sea of norepinephrine, any excess can make insomnia worse and trigger adrenal crashes.

Therefore, a comprehensive recovery plan needs to have components that concurrently address NT imbalance, HPA axis dysregulation, adrenal dysfunction, liver congestion, extracellular matrix pollution, dietary concerns, environmental toxins, etc., to be effective long term.

Wired and Tired

One of the classic signs of NT imbalance in a setting of advanced AFS is a state of being wired and tired. There are several mechanisms that can lead to this state, one of which is NT imbalance. Advanced AFS sufferers are typically in a state of constant fatigue, but yet unable to fall asleep. Those who are able to fall asleep typically wake up after a few hours and are unable to return to sleep easily. As a result, they wake up not being refreshed. Furthermore, many are anxious during the day, followed by energy slumps in the afternoon. When it is time to go to sleep, the body is again wired and tired. It may take a long time to fall asleep, only to be reawakened in a few hours and repeat the cycle again. This can go on for years. Over time, the body becomes weakened. Sleep medications are often required, and over time, dependency and tolerance issues may develop.

In addition to NT imbalance, which is a causative factor in poor sleep, research has shown that much of the wired and tired state is the result of a body flooded in stimulatory catecholamines. Other contributing factors include liver congestion and extracellular matrix pollution. When the body's alarm response is activated because of stress, a state of sympathetic overtone (high norepinephrine typical of early Stage 3C AFS) or reactive sympathetic response (high norepinephrine and epinephrine typical of late Stage 3C AFS) is prevalent. Other symptoms associated with this state include heart palpitations, reactive hypoglycemia, postural orthostatic hypotension, and dizziness.

Normalizing a body in this wired state is a very challenging process because the body is often hypersensitive, so even minute adjustments in NT levels can trigger exaggerated responses in some and paradoxical responses in others. Most issues in resolving this wired and tired state comes from the failure to recognize NT function, dosage errors, improper delivery systems, and a mentality of trying to fix the sleep and anxiety problems rather than looking at them as the consequence of a body in full state of alarm. Because this alarm state is twenty-four seven, successful resolution requires a twenty-four seven approach.

Twenty-Four Hour Neurotransmitter Rhythm and Bias

Our NTs are constantly rebalancing to help us maintain stability twenty-four seven. To be in optimum health, we want to mimic their characteristics during different parts of the day when demands are different. We have clinically identified seven distinct but overlapping phases during the twenty-four hour cycle of the day where the overall NT bias changes.

A comprehensive NT balancing program, to be successful, needs to cover these phases in order to effectively reset the body and return to a state of calm and tranquility. Reestablishing this normal NT rhythm is an attainable goal provided the NT balancing program is attentive to the following seven time-driven phases throughout the day:

- Upon awakening: enhance energy with macro and micronutrition along with a proper breakfast to engage the body for the day's activities. NT focus should be on an excitatory bias to set the body in motion.

- Late morning: sustain energy flow throughout the morning, but keep the body out of anxiety or fatigue, especially during the late morning as energy starts to run low and symptoms of hypoglycemia may surface. The excitatory NT balance should return to a neutral state, avoiding over-excitation.

- Lunch: ensure a proper lunch that provides sufficient sustaining calories for the afternoon along with proper micronutrient supplementation that focuses on continuous energy support, prevention of carbohydrate imbalance that can trigger food coma. The NT balance should be neutral, allowing food from lunch to provide the necessary energy without dependency on excitatory NTs.

- Mid afternoon: support energy flow and prevent energy slumps that can trigger an alarm response with excessive norepinephrine and epinephrine release which can result in adrenal crashes. An afternoon snack may be needed. The NT balance should be slightly excitatory to ensure the body has enough energy to power through the afternoon if a nap is not possible.

- Dinner: gradually down-regulate excitatory NTs through dinner and assure stable assimilation of food without metabolic dysregulation that can trigger inflammation within. The overall NT bias should be slightly inhibitory to set the stage for end-of-day slow down.

- After dinner: transition the body and prepare to unwind as the parasympathetic system takes center stage to carry out the internal housekeeping functions. The NT balance moves closer to the inhibitory bias with acetylcholine as the main NT needed for the parasympathetic nervous system to ensure a mode of rest and digest.

- Middle of the night: supply the body with necessary

inhibitory NTs in order to offset any remaining excitatory stimuli that can prevent the body from entering sleep. Inhibitory NTs are encouraged so the body can fall and stay asleep without metabolic or sympathetic disruptions in the middle of the night.

A battery of natural compounds, dietary and lifestyle modifications are required to support and ensure smooth NT balance throughout the day:

- Exercise: Adrenal restorative exercise, adrenal yoga exercise, adrenal cardiac exercise to help circulation in the morning; adrenal yoga exercise to rebuild internal core strength in midmorning; adrenal restorative exercise in mid afternoon to replenish energy; adrenal liver exercise in the evening to reduce liver stasis; adrenal breathing exercise needs to be incorporated within the exercise routine as well.

- Diet: The proper balance of carbohydrates, protein and fat in meals and snacks with the right frequency and portions to allow fast energy release during the morning, reduced risk of food coma in the early afternoon, avoidance of reactive hypoglycemia throughout the day, adequate caloric reserves before and after exercise, and stable blood sugar during sleep.

Nutritional Supplements Specific for NT Rhythm Modulation

Nutritional supplementation and hormones focused on NTs need to be different for each phase of the day to match the desired goal. Here are some considerations:

- For morning energy and possible midmorning anxiety: magnesium, theanine, GABA, glycine, vitamin B6, pregnenolone, DHEA, vitamin C, glutathione, thyroid support

- For afternoon slumps: hydrolyzed collagen Type 1 and 3, arginine, ribose, pea protein, minerals, glutamine, holy basil, milk thistle, chromium, glutamine

- For early evening anxiety: magnesium, theanine, taurine, zinc, selenium, fish oil, 5-HTP, low dose GABA

- For sleep onset insomnia: niacin, magnesium, 5-HTP, GABA, valerian root, passionflower, melatonin, progesterone, arginine, vitamin D, fish oil

- For sleep maintenance insomnia: time-release chromium polynicotinate, 5-HTP, niacinamide, magnesium, taurine, 5- HTP, passion flower, and melatonin.

Additional organ specific nutrients to support NT balance can be deployed. They include:

- Liver support: liposomal glutathione, fermented milk thistle, NAC, lipoic acid, calcium d-glucarate

- Anti-inflammatory support: quercetin, bromelain, fish oil, vitamin D, holy basil

- Calming support: GABA, 5-HTP, theanine, magnesium, taurine, niacin, valerian root, melatonin, phosphatidylserine, arginine, glycine, inositol

- Excitation support: tyrosine, minerals, vitamin B12, DHEA, thyroid glandular, adrenal cortex, pregnenolone

- Adrenal support: vitamin C, mineral ascorbate,

ascorbylpalmitate, pantethine (B5), pregnenolone, DHEA

- Thyroid support: zinc, selenium, thyroid glandular, iodine, kelp
- Extracellular matrix support: ingestible clay, marine minerals, essential oil, activated charcoal, and germanium

It should be understood that NT balancing is a highly technical aspect of nutritional medicine. It requires in-depth clinical experience due to its complexity and lack of well correlated scientific clinical markers. The rather simplistic approach of simple replenishment of what appears to be depleted based on laboratory testing seldom works and in fact can worsen the overall condition over time.

A comprehensive plan is necessarily tedious, time consuming and all encompassing because we are dealing with chemicals that have wide ranging effects throughout the body. Most NT imbalances have underlying root causes that need to be addressed first to effect long-term healing. This is especially true when NT imbalance occurs in a setting of AFS. Fortunately, once NTs are stabilized, the recovery program can be discontinued. The younger the sufferer, the faster is the recovery. Unfortunately, most people tend to underestimate or are unaware of the long-term negative consequences of NT imbalance. Many healthcare practitioners are not well educated in this aspect of medicine. Sufferers stumble through many trial and error attempts, which can worsen the overall condition.

Key Points to Remember:

Neurotransmitters (NTs) are the chemical messengers used to send signals throughout our nervous system. They have a wide variety of functions encompassing almost everything that happens in our body.

There are two major classes of NTs, excitatory and inhibitory. As their names imply, excitatory NTs promote alertness and activity while inhibitory NTs makes you feel good, cause sleepiness and prevent overexcitation.

Imbalances in NT levels can be caused by a variety of factors including poor diet, environmental toxins and stress. In advanced AFS, neurotransmitter imbalance causes a state of being wired and tired, where sufferers may be anxious and tired at the same time during the day, and find themselves unable to relax and rest well at night.

NT repletion medications can often build dependency and resistance, and end up depleting the NT instead, exacerbating the imbalance. Instead, long term NT repletion can be achieved by providing the body the necessary building blocks to rebuild and rebalance NT levels on its own.

This is a challenge in advanced AFS, as supplementation with these building blocks can be too stimulatory, trigger paradoxical reactions, and stress the body causing a crash.

For proper rebalancing of NTs in an AFS setting, many moving parts need to be addressed to slowly and steadily move the body along the recovery path. This process is necessarily time consuming as any stumbles can set back the body and make the road to recovery even longer.

Chapter 4

Severe Insomnia: Biological Rhythm Disruption

Advanced Adrenal Fatigue Syndrome (AFS) invariably is accompanied by some form of sleep disruption clinically. Many report being unable to fall asleep as well as frequent awakenings during the sleep cycle. Without a good night's rest, the body's ability to restore itself is compromised. Waking up unrefreshed is a common complaint. As more energy is required for normal daily activities, the body's energy pool drains; morning and afternoon slumps are a common occurrence. With each day the body gets weaker and experiences more fatigue. Heroic efforts are often used to force the body to sleep at night. This usually fails in advanced AFS because the body's natural biological rhythm is disrupted. Repairing such dysfunction requires a 24 hour daily cycle approach, not simply taking sleeping pills at bedtime. These may facilitate sleep, but not do anything to repair the biological rhythm and bodily functions. Here are some signs and symptoms of biological rhythm disruption:

- Inability to fall asleep
- Waking up in the middle of the night without being able to return to sleep
- Waking up unrefreshed
- Mid-morning slumps
- Mid-afternoon slumps
- Second wind in the early evening

- Inability to sleep when going to bed early
- Sensitivity to drugs and nutritional supplements
- Mood instability
- Being easily irritated
- Feeling more alert in the evening than during the day
- Coffee helps the sleep
- Menstrual cycle disruptions

Biological Rhythm Disruptions and Adrenal Fatigue Syndrome

Our biological rhythm (BR) refers to the natural rhythm that certain bodily functions and activities follow. This includes our body temperature, level of alertness, sleep schedule, and endocrine activity. Our BR usually repeats in predictable cycles of time. The menstrual cycle, for example, occurs every twenty-eight days. Rhythms that follow a twenty-four hour cycle are often referred to as circadian rhythms, such as our sleep–wake cycle. Our brain helps maintain and control our internal clock that regulates these rhythms.

There are external factors that can have an influence on our BR; for example, sunlight and certain drugs like caffeine can affect our sleep schedule. Disorders can also develop when our natural BR is interrupted or disturbed. They include:

- Sleep disorders, insomnia
- Mood disorders, depression and seasonal affective disorder
- Shift-work disorders
- Jet lag

- Metabolic imbalances

As AFS progresses through its four stages from mild to severe, BR disruptions tend to be more pronounced. Most advanced AFS suffers therefore have severe insomnia. In advanced stages of AFS, many sufferers are simply unable to fall asleep (also called "sleep onset insomnia" or SOI) or stay asleep (also called 'sleep maintenance insomnia" or SMI) because they feel both wired and tired . In very severe cases, catnaps are the only way the patient can get any sleep, which means they can end up being sleep deprived for days at a time. Scientific research has revealed that a great many of these cases are caused by BR disruptions secondary to hormonal and neurotransmitter (NT) dysregulation.

In this chapter we examine the role BR plays in insomnia in a setting of advanced AFS and suggests natural approaches and solutions when sleep aids have failed.

Biological Rhythm Basics

Chronobiology is an area of biology examining periodic or cyclic occurrences in living organisms and their synchronization with natural rhythms. These cycles are called biological rhythms (BR). Research in this area involves the study of other fields such as neurology, space medicine, sleep medicine, endocrinology and psychology. This is not the same as biorhythm, which is really just a pseudoscience attempting to explain cyclic variations in the behavior of humans based on emotional and physiological cycles, and has nothing to do with chronobiology.

The duration and timing of biological activity cycles in organisms varies among the many essential biological processes. The most vital rhythm in chronobiology would be the circadian rhythm. This is roughly a twenty-four hour cycle indicated by physiological processes in nearly all living organisms. Circadian rhythm controls:

- Endocrine rhythms
- Sleep timing
- Performance
- Behavior

All this is regulated and controlled by the circadian clock, which is a collection of nerves in the region of the brain known as the hypothalamus. Other forms of biological rhythm include:

- Tidal Rhythms—Often seen in marine life, they follow a roughly 12.4-hour cycle from low tide to high tide and back.

- Infradian Rhythms—These cycles last longer than twenty-four hours, such as the yearly migration of birds or the reproduction cycles of certain animals and, of course, the human female menstrual cycle.

- Gene Oscillations—Certain genes are expressed more during specific hours of the day.

- Ultradian Rhythms—Cycles lasting less than twenty-four hours, as the REM sleep cycle that lasts ninety minutes, or the three-hour cycle that produces growth hormones.

Biological Rhythm Disruptions

Animals, plants, cyanobacteria and fungi have all been observed having biological rhythms. Even though these different BR are internally controlled, there are some external factors that can influence their regularity.

Factors that can alter the BR greatly include changes in light brought about by seasonal transitions, changes in work schedules affecting sleeping hours, severe or unrelenting stress, jet lag, toxic overload, neurotransmitter imbalances, and receptor site disorders. The factors also include chronic conditions such as dysregulation of the neuroendocrine system or AFS, dysregulation of the autonomic nervous system, which includes an overabundance of norepinephrine (known as sympathetic overtone), overabundance of epinephrine (known as reactive sympathetic response), and polluted extracellular matrix. These factors also include glucose intolerance, metabolic syndrome, reactive hypoglycemia, excessive metabolic build-up from liver congestion, improper detoxification, reaction to retoxification, unresolved stealth infection, aging, weight loss, pregnancy, OAT axis disruption, HPA axis dysregulation, paradoxical results from medication and/or natural remedies including herbs, excessive or prolonged use of antibiotics, pH imbalance, caffeine, severe infection, and weak constitution.

Just about any condition that brings about an imbalance in internal homeostasis can disrupt the BR. The onset can be gradual or acute. The classic presenting complaint indicating a disrupted BR is insomnia. Some have reported a case of sudden onset of insomnia after experiencing an extremely stressful event or after taking a course of antibiotics. Others have reported a gradual onset that spans months when their sleep pattern begins to become slightly disrupted and gradually worsens over time.

Disorders in BR can affect sleep–wake cycles, body temperature, the release of hormones and other vital bodily functions. They have been associated with:

- Sleep disorders such as insomnia

- Mood disorders such as depression, anxiety and bipolar disorder

- Obesity

- Metabolic syndrome

- Diabetes

- Seasonal affective disorder, a form of depression

Since very few clinicians are looking for biological rhythm disruptions when examining a patient complaining of insomnia, it is hardly ever recognized as a problem until the BR disruption becomes severe. This is often the case when associated with advanced AFS.

The most common presenting complaint from those suffering from BR disruption is severe insomnia. Instead of trying to determine the root cause of sleep disturbance and restoring proper BR as the ultimate long-term solution, most try to self-navigate at first with sleep aids, such as melatonin or over-the-counter antihistamines. When the sleep aids fail, stronger medications are taken. This usually works for a while, but eventually the body develops tolerance as well as dependency.

To make matters worse, most sufferers of chronic insomnia invariably have low energy during the day. They are frequently prescribed stimulants to increase energy to help them make it through the day after the effects of coffee diminish. These compounds include DHEA, testosterone, vitamin B12, pregnenolone, and various herbs like green tea, rhodiola, maca, ashwagandha, and ginseng. Coffee intake has usually already become a habit by now. Patients are usually hyped up throughout the day and later stay wired and unable to calm down and relax at bedtime.

Inevitably, stronger prescription sleep medication is used

to induce sleep. Without solving the underlying BR disruption, sleep forced on by medication only lasts a few hours and sufferers now awaken frequently in the middle of the night unable to return to sleep. Those with weak constitutions may have metabolic disruptions in the middle of the night because of BR imbalances. They awaken after a few hours of sleep experiencing heart palpitations, perspiration, and anxiety.

In severe cases, visits to the ER with extensive workups only result in being pronounced well and sent home. Typically sufferers wake up in the middle of the night and are not able to return to sleep easily, and when morning dawns they do not feel at all refreshed or ready to take on the new day. They drag themselves through the day only to repeat the same insomniac cycle the following night.

Left unattended, BR disruptions become more severe and intractable chronic insomnia becomes the norm. Many resort to only taking catnaps during the day and remain awake throughout the night. By now, prescription sleep medications don't continue to work as well and many have reached their maximum dosage. The patient is also typically maxed out on stimulants during the day. With no other options, their doctor concedes defeat and abandons the patient. By now their BR is severely disrupted. Fortunately, this clinical picture is not a frequent occurrence as it represents extreme situations. Unfortunately, sufferers that do reach this state are left with no options and nowhere to turn for help. To restore BR, we first need to review how our internal master clock is involved.

The Master Clock

There happens to be a master clock inside our brain that coordinates all our biological cycles to make sure they are synchronized. This is made up of a grouping of nerve cells called the suprachiasmatic nucleus (SCN). It contains approximately 20,000 nerve cells and can be found in the hypothalamus. This is where the production of melatonin is controlled, which is the hormone that helps to bring on sleep. The SCN can be found right above the optic nerves. The optic nerves send messages from the eyes to our brain, which means the SCN gets information regarding incoming light. At night there is less light so the SCN instructs the brain to produce more melatonin to make us sleepy. Therefore more melatonin is produced and secreted at nighttime and ebbs during daytime. The presence of melatonin gives the brain the information it needs about the length of the night.

Neurotransmitters play a very big part in how the SCN functions in our brain. The strength of our circadian rhythms depends on how accurately our biological clock is functioning and how well it is integrated into the actions of the thousands of separate cellular clocks contained within. Neurotransmitters are working in all areas of this system, during the input of information, within the clock itself, and in the efferent output needed to inform the body's processes.

The phase markers used to measure the timing of the BR of mammals are:

• Core body temperature

• Heart rate

• Melatonin

• Cortisol

• Production of red blood cells

Seven Clinical Temporal Biological Rhythms

Our daily circadian rhythm can be broken down clinically into seven sub-rhythms that follow one another.

Awakening Rhythm

This occurs from 6 to 9 a.m. We stop secreting melatonin by about 7:30 a.m. It is the body's natural way of saying it is time to get up. To facilitate the awakening process, cortisol, an important anti-stress hormone secreted from the adrenal glands, rises during the early morning hours. Cortisol levels are at their peak around 8:30 a.m.

Our heart rate and blood pressure rises as well in the early morning hours while our output of norepinephrine increases. This allows us to stand up from a horizontal position and move around physically so we can begin our day productively.

Our GI tract also has its active phase after awakening. The large intestine acts to let go physically as well as emotionally. Most can expect a bowel movement by around 9 a.m. However, a much better time for this would be before 7 a.m.

Morning Rhythm

This occurs from 9 a.m. to noon. Most adults are busy at work during this time, with a draw on our brainpower and physical reserves, depending on our activity. This is when our testosterone is at its highest output, which means we are on full alert by 10 a.m. Traditional Chinese medicine claims the spleen pulls the needed nutrients from our food, transforming it into energy that is sent to other organ systems throughout our body during this time frame. If we experience bloating after meals, loose stool, low energy and crave sweets, these symptoms indicate an imbalance. People who are weak or have AFS may become tired and anxious in the late morning hours. Typically, BR disruption tends to be more pronounced from 11 a.m. to noon, with symptoms indicating an imbalance including:

- Heart palpitations
- Shortness of breath
- Cold hands and feet
- Insomnia
- Anxiety

Lunch Rhythm

This occurs from noon to 2 p.m. Most people look forward to lunch as a time to replenish their energy. After lunch, our small intestine starts working to help food assimilation. If the person has ingested too many carbohydrates at lunch, causing metabolic dysfunction, they could experience a food coma and start feeling sleepy after the meal.

If you have not consumed enough water throughout the morning, you will likely feel dehydrated during this part of the day. When you are out of balance, certain physical conditions may develop which can include bloating with gas or even vomiting and a duodenal ulcer.

Afternoon Rhythm

This occurs from 2 to 6 p.m. You are likely to experience a mid-afternoon slump in energy and focus and this typically occurs between the hours of 3 to 5 p.m.

The key is mid-afternoon between 2 to 4 p.m. After the immediate energy surge has exhausted itself, as in the case of AFS, fatigue returns. Your blood sugar levels may be within the normal range, but you feel lethargic. Those with metabolic issues may experience reactive hypoglycemia. During this time of day you can easily feel a drop in energy, especially if you have not consumed enough water and are dehydrated. When this imbalance occurs you may feel a burning sensation when urinating, develop a yeast infection or even urinary incontinence.

Our body is most coordinated at about 2 p.m. This is when our body's cardiovascular system is performing most efficiently. Our muscles have warmed up and our level of stress is decreasing as the day's end approaches. Our greatest muscle strength occurs around 5 p.m. This is the time of day when people are least likely to have a heart attack while exercising as the body can better handle the physical strain.

Dinner Rhythm

This occurs from 6 to 9 p.m., around dinnertime. The body reaches its highest temperature at 7 p.m. while the neurotransmitters responsible for carrying out the day's activities are still going strong. Cortisol has been gradually declining since mid-morning and continues.

As light begins to dim, a process known as Dim Light Melatonin Onset (DLMO) begins around 9 p.m. and can be detected in blood or saliva. Melatonin's most prominent metabolite can be detected in the morning urine. DLMO and the midpoint of melatonin blood or saliva presence are commonly used as circadian markers.

Sleep Onset Rhythm

This occurs from 10 p.m. to 2 a.m. You are now suppressing any bowel movement as you begin your sleep cycle. During sleep, you cycle back and forth between REM and non-REM periods of sleep. Your lowest cortisol levels occur around midnight.

You begin with non-REM sleep then you experience a shorter time of REM sleep. The cycle then repeats. During REM sleep you will typically have dreams.

Non-REM sleep occurs in three different phases. Each phase lasts from five to fifteen minutes. You experience all phases before achieving REM sleep.

- Phase 1 – Although your eyes are shut, it's still easy to awaken you. You will be in this phase for five to ten minutes.

- Phase 2 – You are in a light slumber. Your heart rate has slowed down and your body temperature has dropped. Your body is preparing for a deep sleep.

- Phase 3 – This is when you are in a deep sleep. It's more difficult to awaken you during this phase. If someone does wake you up, you will be disoriented for several minutes.

During the phases of deep non-REM sleep, your body repairs and regrows bone and muscle tissue, while the immune system becomes stronger.

Rapid Eye Movement (REM) sleep is a stage of sleep when your eyes are quickly moving in different directions. This doesn't occur during non-REM periods of sleep. Typically, people enter REM sleep around ninety minutes after first falling asleep. Each of the later REM sleep phases lasts longer, and the last one of the night can last up to an hour. Your breathing and heart rate becomes quicker.

During REM sleep your brain increases in activity so you are able to have more intense dreams.

Most people, when allowed to sleep for as long as they want, will sleep for approximately nine hours. Age does affect sleep however. As you age, you tend to sleep more lightly and not get as much deep sleep. Newborns sleep twice as much as adults do. There are differences in the individual sleep requirements of people, and studies on twins reveal these differences may be partly genetic.

Your body should be completely immersed in your sleep cycles as the night continues on, reaching your deepest sleep around 2 a.m.

Sleep Maintenance Rhythm

This occurs from 2 to 6 a.m. The body is now on automatic cruise control, resting and rejuvenating. The lowest body temperature is reached at about 5 a.m. Cortisol levels start rising at around 2 to 3 a.m. with levels continuing to climb throughout the balance of the night until we awaken in the morning. Our level of alertness is at its lowest from 4 to 6 a.m.

Metabolic dysfunctions such as sugar imbalances, excessive stress, anger and resentment can cause excessive neurotransmitter (NT) release, waking you up. If you're not sleeping at this time, you can quickly become deficient. You may find that you wake up between 2 to 4 a.m. if you have repressed anger or long standing resentment. According to traditional Chinese medicine, liver cleansing also takes place during this time. BR disruptions during this phase can lead to liver and extracellular matrix (ECM) congestion, meaning that the body is unable to process its metabolites efficiently. Other symptoms of liver and ECM imbalance include irregular menstruation, anemia, chronic fatigue, and headache. Symptoms of liver imbalances include irregular menstruation, anemia, chronic fatigue, and headache. According to traditional Chinese medicine, liver cleansing takes place during this time. BR disruptions during this phase can lead to liver and extracellular matrix congestion.

Severe Insomnia—the Classic BR Dysfunction

According to the World Health Organization, a full 40 percent of the population worldwide suffers from some form of sleep disorder. Along with disruptions in sleep, or the inability to sleep, these circadian rhythm disturbances can change our body mass index as well as cause behavioral disorders.

Fundamentally we process incoming information on two different levels. Our conscious mind processes information in a serial manner, which is fairly slow. However, because we are aware and able to focus, we are able to act voluntarily, performing functions like problem solving, moving our muscles, and communicating verbally with others.

When we are unconscious our mind is still processing incoming information and we can perform tasks that are familiar to us automatically. In this state, our senses and neural pathways continue to rapidly register stimuli on multiple tracks simultaneously without us being consciously aware or knowing that all of this is going on. This is how we digest food and regulate sleep. Because our body continues to run due to our autonomic nervous system, we are thus able to maintain our BR phases throughout the day, making adjustments to stay in sync with our various activities, whether we are awake or asleep.

Our biological clock is very sensitive to internal and external cues, so it can become easily desynchronized from a number of different factors:

- Social or lifestyle factors like shift work

- Mutations in our clock's genes leading to aberrant regulation

- Impaired or desynchronized neurotransmitters

We examined neurotransmitters themselves in detail in the previous chapter. Here we will explore how our molecular clock regulates the levels of neurotransmitters in our system, including the level of serotonin. A malfunctioning clock can lead to impaired neurotransmission. The reverse is true in that impaired neurotransmission may affect our molecular clock's synchronization. Whether a malfunctioning molecular clock is cause or effect is up for debate. However, many psychiatric conditions and disorders, including depression, bipolar disorder and schizophrenia are linked to disruptions in circadian rhythms.

When psychiatric disorders are treated with pharmaceutical drugs, the medications prescribed often entail restoring balance to the patient's dysfunctional neurotransmission systems. However a better outcome might possibly be achieved by addressing the dysfunction also existing in the patient's molecular clock.

If our neurotransmitters are disrupted or dysregulated, combined with a neuroendocrine dysregulation such as that of AFS, our health can suffer due to the normal biological rhythms being disrupted, with symptoms such as:

- Anxiety

- Moodiness

- Being easily irritated

- Tendency toward bipolar behavior

- Mild anger

- Panic attacks

- Feeling wired but tired at the same time

- Insomnia

Eight Chemical Imbalances that Result in BR Disruption and Insomnia

1. Serotonin Deficiency: Serotonin is an extremely important neurotransmitter, often referred to as the master neurotransmitter. Serotonin plays a very important part in regulating our sleep–wake cycles over the course of twenty-four hours. It links the rhythmic activity occurring in the basal forebrain and the preoptic area to the circadian rhythm being signaled by the suprachiasmatic nucleus (SCN). Serotonin essentially links our sleep–wake cycles with our body's natural twenty-four hour cycle, synchronizing them.

The symptoms that occur when someone is deficient in serotonin are:

- Anxiety

- Depression

- Excessive worrying

- Panic attacks

- Obsessive thoughts

- Premenstrual syndrome

- Fatigue

- Heat intolerance

- Fibromyalgia

When serotonin levels are abnormally low there is an inadequate supply and certainly not enough surplus to convert to melatonin. This results in difficulty falling asleep at night, commonly referred to as night owl syndrome. This is more common than having difficulty staying asleep, although someone can suffer from both. When someone is experiencing excessive worry and obsessive thoughts, these alone make it difficult to fall asleep and make being awake very unpleasant. This condition is often genetically passed and of a longstanding nature, although it may become more problematic over time.

In addition to the symptoms listed above, when someone is suffering from a depletion of serotonin they also frequently display the following symptoms:

- Craving carbs and alcohol in the afternoon and/or evening premature awakening
- Negative thoughts or frame of mind
- Low self-esteem
- Perfectionism
- Rage and anger
- Controlling and obsessive behaviors
- Phobias like fear of heights, snakes, small spaces, etc.

5-HTP is the biological precursor to serotonin. 5-HTP can be used to increase serotonin in the body. When you first begin supplementing with 5-HTP you should take a very low dose, gradually working your way up. The right dose depends on the individual, their needs and what their body can tolerate. The correct amount can vary from 50 to 300 mg per day in divided doses.

Our bodies maintain a balance in terms of serotonin and cortisol production. The more serotonin we have present, the more cortisol our body produces and vice versa. Our adrenal glands produce cortisol and as such contain receptors that can sense how much serotonin is in our bloodstream at any given time. When the adrenal glands are exposed to serotonin, they release cortisol into our bloodstream. This means that by taking 5-HTP and increasing the levels of serotonin, you can increase the body's cortisol levels. This may not be beneficial for those with AFS, depending on their stage. Because 5-HTP can raise cortisol, 5-HTP usage should be carefully considered if cortisol is high as it is in early stages of AFS. Most with advanced AFS have low cortisol so 5-HTP can be helpful in such cases. Large doses of 5-HTP, however, may cause nausea on an empty stomach, so 5-HTP is best taken with a snack or beverage. These symptoms may only occur at certain points in the day, e.g., at bedtime and not during the day, during the night or in the early hours of the morning when taken.

When taken in extremely high doses, 5-HTP can cause serotonin toxicity or serotonin syndrome, and this can literally be fatal. Serotonin syndrome can occur if you are taking prescription medications, particularly antidepressants that affect the body's level of serotonin. The greatest risk occurs if you are taking two or more drugs and/or supplements together that influence serotonin. The most commonly prescribed class of antidepressants, which work by increasing serotonin, is the serotonin reuptake inhibitors (SSRIs). These include Celexa, Lexapro, Paxil, Prozac, and Zoloft. The condition is more likely to occur when you first start a medicine or upon increasing the dose.

L-theanine is another amino acid and precursor to serotonin. It helps in the production of GABA and dopamine and is related to another nonessential amino acid, glutamine. It is considered to be psychoactive since it has the ability to penetrate the blood-brain barrier. L-theanine is converted to several useful calming and mood-elevating substances in the brain, including GABA, allowing one to indirectly supplement the brain with GABA.

Because L-theanine is known for helping to relieve stress and provide relaxation, it is used in some sleep remedies in conjunction with low dose 5-HTP, GABA, melatonin, and calming herbs like passion flower and valerian root.

Recommended dosage of theanine: Take 100 to 400 mg in divided doses daily. Those with advanced AFS need to be on alert for paradoxical reactions. Stop supplementation if this occurs.

2. Melatonin Deficiency: The pineal gland produces melatonin, which is thought to influence our body's internal processes, helping all the bodily systems work in a coordinated manner. When the internal systems become disorganized or out of sync the body becomes more vulnerable to disease. The levels of melatonin in the bloodstream fluctuate throughout the day, but surge during nighttime when it's dark outside and it's time for sleep.

The common symptoms of a melatonin deficiency are:

- Disturbed sleep

- Sleep onset insomnia

- Night owl behavior

Melatonin has become popular among those seeking a natural sleep aid. When taking melatonin supplements you need to be careful to take the correct dose. There are those that can absorb and assimilate melatonin very easily and can benefit from just a fraction of a milligram. Others need to take 50 mg to achieve the desired effect. The resulting effect is not at all linear so a period of trial and error is needed by an experienced clinician to determine the proper dosage. People experiencing a hangover in the morning after taking melatonin should try taking it two hours before bedtime rather than right at bedtime.

Melatonin does not work in the same manner as a sleeping pill or even 5-HTP because melatonin supplements will only be effective in producing a sedative effect if the levels of melatonin in the user are low to begin with.

Melatonin is a hormone naturally produced in the body from serotonin, but since 5-HTP is a precursor for serotonin, 5-HTP can also increase the levels of melatonin in the body. A certain level of serotonin is required as a primer to start the production of melatonin. For some, a threshold level of serotonin is also needed in the body to relax enough to fall asleep. Melatonin produced after the onset of sleep helps the person remain asleep.

When your body is not producing enough melatonin, you can suffer from mood disorders, anxiety, insomnia, lowered basal body temperature, a suppressed immune system, and an elevated estrogen/progesterone ratio. When your body is producing too much melatonin you can suffer from low thyroid and adrenal function, seasonal affective disorder (SAD), hypotension, and a lowered estrogen/progesterone ratio.

3. Melatonin and Serotonin Imbalance: Melatonin and serotonin work together in sync. Serotonin is the powerful neurotransmitter from which melatonin is derived and is involved in a number of physiological processes which are central to our health, including the regulation of blood-pressure, our perception of pain, as well as some neuropsychological functions like memory, mood and appetite. Just as with melatonin, serotonin levels affect a variety of endocrine activities performed by the pituitary gland, the hypothalamus and others.

For the most part, serotonin and melatonin do not act in the body together or at the same time. Melatonin is actively involved at night and serotonin does its work during the daytime. Both are involved in moderating endocrine functions, but serotonin seems to have a negative influence on the cardiovascular system when its levels in the bloodstream are too high. There have been cases of this causing a narrowing of blood vessels and blood clotting as well as other adverse effects. Unlike with melatonin, the levels of serotonin in our body do not decrease as we get older, but increases relative to other neurotransmitters and hormones.

Scientists who have studied aging and the elderly think that this imbalance between melatonin and serotonin, which is age-related, may be as important a factor in the aging processes as the lack of melatonin, especially as it relates to heart disease.

Without enough melatonin acting as a scavenger for free radicals during the night, blood vessels may become more damaged, which stimulates the release of additional serotonin.

Research has revealed that people suffering from severe depression are lacking enough serotonin, norepinephrine and dopamine, three essential neurotransmitters actively used by the brain. Therefore, the link between serotonin and melatonin, along with their governance by the body clock might explain the depression felt by those suffering from seasonal affective disorder (SAD).

4. GABA Deficiency: GABA is a powerful neurotransmitter that performs an inhibitory function, often being called Nature's Valium. When the body is producing high levels of GABA, this indicates the body is experiencing excitatory overload due to the higher demand for GABA to balance out the excess excitatory neurotransmitters like glutamate. Low levels of GABA are linked with hypothalamus-pituitary axis feedback dysfunction and adrenal distress.

Symptoms of a GABA deficiency include:

- Feeling uptight

- Being burned out

- Feeling overwhelmed

- Sore muscles

If GABA is deficient in the body, it can be supplemented by using a supplemental form of GABA. Each of us may have different amounts of GABA in the brain that is considered normal. There is no medical testing standard that determines whether GABA activity is too high or too low. However, excessive use of street drugs, alcohol, and prescription drugs are associated with low GABA activity and a state of excitation.

GABA's primary function is to neutralize epinephrine (also

known as adrenaline). A deficiency in GABA can combine with a deficiency in serotonin and melatonin or cause problems with sleep on its own. This is when muscle tension and other symptoms of GABA deficiency, like being stressed, can disrupt sleep. The primary symptoms associated with this deficiency are feeling overwhelmed, overstressed without the ability to loosen up and relax, and feeling burned out, with tense or stiff muscles. When people with a GABA deficiency take sleep medications they may have panic attacks. People with this condition are likely to respond best when they take benzodiazepines. If GABA deficiency is suspected, 100 to 500 mg of GABA may be considered. You can take this with or in place of melatonin or tryptophan. Avoid taking high doses of 750 mg or more at one time or it may cause anxiety instead. For those who do not respond to GABA, you may want to try I-theanine, which can result in a calming effect.

Taurine. Taurine is an amino acid that calms the nervous system by facilitating the production of the neurotransmitter GABA. By helping to raise GABA levels, taurine allows the body to manage anxiety so that your thoughts don't go spiraling out of control and you don't experience the associated cortisol and epinephrine spikes seen in AFS.

Take taurine together with magnesium for better sleep. Together these nutrients also abolish stress, calm the nervous system and improve mood. Deficiency in magnesium or taurine poses a risk for depression and poor motivation.

5. Excessive High Cortisol: Cortisol has a very interesting and distinctive circadian rhythm. It reaches its lowest levels around midnight, then begins rising around 2 to 3 a.m., reaching its peak around 8:30 a.m., at which time it begins slowly decreasing back to the lowest point, which completes the cycle in twenty-four hours.

The regulation of cortisol release, or glucocorticoids, is determined by the action of the HPA axis. The HPA axis receives information coming in from the central pacemaker that controls circadian release of the corticotropin-releasing hormone (CRH) going into the paraventricular nucleus. This is also set off by emotional and physical stressors. The CRH triggers the release of the adrenocorticotropic hormones (ACTH) coming from the corticotropin cells located in the anterior pituitary, followed by the glucocorticoid cortisol coming from the adrenal cortex. Cortisol then exerts its inhibitory effects at hypothalamic and pituitary levels, performing a classic negative feedback loop, although the SCN receives no feedback.

Our adrenal gland has its own circadian clock whose job it is to set specific intervals of time when it most efficiently responds to ACTH. The splanchnic nerve regulates all of this. Genes for the clock are expressed in a rhythm in the zona fasciculate and zonaglomerulosa, as well as all the pathways characteristically used by the adrenal gland; like for the production of the catecholamines and steroid metabolism. The expression of the clock genes by the adrenal gland reveals a six-hour phase delay related to the SCN, which is primarily induced through the SCN without any associated activation of the HPA axis. This expression of genes goes along with the rhythmic secretion of brain and plasma cortisol.

A number of separate episodes of cortisol secretion occur over the span of a twenty-four hour day totaling four different and unequal temporal phases. These phases are experienced as: a period of little secretory activity, during which time there is negligible cortisol secretion and occurs four hours before the onset of sleep and two hours after the onset of sleep; a preliminary episode of nocturnal secretions around the third to fifth hours of sleep; a primary phase of secretions with three to five episodes happening during the sixth to eight hours of sleep which continue through to the first hour of being awake; and four to nine intermittent secretory activity episodes while awake that occur in the second to twelfth hours of being awake.

In the early stages of AFS, a state of high cortisol output exists. This can even occur long after the events causing the stress have been resolved or with long standing perceived stress and not actual stress. If cortisol disturbance occurs at night, when the levels are supposed to be at their lowest, the type of insomnia experienced is an alert, which feels like your body is ready to do something. It is a state of hypervigilance and agitation, or you might feel shocked or suddenly startled awake in the middle of the night. Both SOI and SMI can be expected.

Phosphatidylserine (PS) is a natural compound with cortisol lowering capabilities. It can repair the cortisol receptors in the hypothalamus that are damaged by chronically high cortisol. PS can be effectively used to calm elevated levels of cortisol at night and help induce sleep. However, it is common to have paradoxical responses in advanced stages of AFS. The weaker the body is, the higher prevalence of paradoxical reaction.

Other options include phosphorylated serine which seems to have a much stronger ability to lower cortisol levels. Bioactive hydrolyzed peptide is another effective supplement. Holy basil, magnolia bark and reishi may also help. To treat the kidneys and adrenal glands, acupuncture and/or Chinese herbs can be considered, especially in cases where cortisol levels are high during day and night.

Do not take supplements that tend to be stimulating or are known to raise cortisol levels, such as ashwagandha, licorice, maca, green tea, rhodiola. L-tyrosine is a stimulating amino acid that converts into norepinephrine and epinephrine and exacerbates insomnia caused by high cortisol.

If benzodiazepines are used as sleep aids and an addiction develops, these need to be maintained or tapered off while making sure all of the recommended nutrients are provided, guided by medical professionals.

6. Catecholamine Overload: There are three catecholamines in our body: dopamine, norepinephrine (neurotransmitter for

the sympathetic nervous system), and epinephrine. When your system is overloaded with catecholamines you will experience the following symptoms:

- Heart palpitations
- Fast heart rate when resting
- Anxiety
- Racing thoughts
- Dizziness when standing
- Inability to fall asleep
- Waking frequently with a fast heart rate
- Vivid dreams
- Nightmares

Dopamine is the neurotransmitter that helps us concentrate and focus. When the ratio between dopamine and serotonin is out of balance you will typically have difficulty focusing, remembering things like where you left your keys and you may find yourself daydreaming. Dopamine is involved in controlling the brain's reward and pleasure center as well as playing a role in regulating our sleep.

Researchers have found that dopamine receptors appear in the pineal gland only towards the end of nighttime. When dopamine interacts with its own receptors, the effects of norepinephrine are stopped, which causes the production and the release of melatonin to become lower. This signals the brain that it is time to wake up.

Norepinephrine acts as an excitatory neurotransmitter in the body to stimulate body processes. When norepinephrine and epinephrine activate the body's sympathetic nervous system, our ability to concentrate and focus is affected. When levels of norepinephrine are elevated, we can experience insomnia, irritability, racing thoughts, headaches, feeling wired, and anxiousness.

Norepinephrine is chemically derived from dopamine and carries out its functions by attaching to the receptors for dopamine in cell membranes. Chronic stress puts the HPA hormonal axis in overdrive as AFS progresses. In advanced AFS, the HPA axis becomes overburdened and disrupted. The body then activates the sympathetic nervous system (SNS) to keep in high gear and handle stress by releasing norepinephrine. A chronically high norepinephrine is called "sympathetic overtone." The body is constantly on alert, unable to relax. Sleep becomes difficult even though the body is tired, with frequent awakenings a few hours later as the body is repeatedly put on alert by excessive norepinephrine. Many common street drugs work by mimicking norepinephrine in the brain and causing a mental high.

Epinephrine is derived from norepinephrine and is another excitatory neurotransmitter, but this one is involved in our body's fight or flight protective response. Epinephrine regulates certain brain functions like heart rate, blood pressure and metabolism.

When we have lower levels of epinephrine in our body, we can experience depression, fatigue, burnout, dizziness, and poor recovery from illness, as well as inability to deal with stress.

If the adrenal glands are overstimulated for a long period of time, as occurs in advanced stages of AFS, this can set off a massive release of epinephrine as the body becomes engaged in the fight or flight response. The symptoms include panic attacks, nervousness, a sense of impending doom, atrial fibrillation and postural orthostatic tachycardia. Visits to emergency rooms are common, but test results are unremarkable and suffers are simply sent home to rest.

7. Glutamate Overload: Glutamate is an excitatory neurotransmitter. This one, to a large extent, is involved in learning

114

and memory.

Symptoms associated with elevated levels of glutamate include depression, panic attacks, anxiety, headaches, and irritability.

Symptoms associated with low levels of glutamate include lethargy, depression, memory loss, and insomnia.

Glutamate is intimately involved with GABA and glutamine in a process that balances the level of each in the body. As a precursor to both glutamate and GABA, glutamine is the gatekeeper determining how much of these NTs is produced.

If the body is excited, anxious or in a severe inflammatory state, more GABA than glutamate is produced from glutamine to calm the body in theory. Unfortunately, inflammation can disrupt the cycle and instead produce excess glutamate. It is not unusual to see a variety of paradoxical reactions when supplementing glutamine, especially in advanced AFS.

Generally speaking, controlling glutamate intake can help prevent over excitation. For example, monosodium glutamate (MSG) is a flavor enhancer, often used in Chinese food, that should be avoided.

Care must be taken to lower glutamate intake as it is a major component of protein rich foods like meat, eggs, poultry, milk, cheese, and fish. Glutamate or glutamic acid is also ubiquitous in grain, beans, vegetables, mushrooms, fruits, nuts, and sea vegetables. Foods with high levels of glutamate include Parmesan cheese, soy sauce, walnuts, fresh tomato juice, grape juice, peas, mushrooms, broccoli, tomatoes, oysters and corn.

BR Rebalancing Principles

BR disruptions may present classically as insomnia, but the underlying circadian disruption is a twenty-four-seven phenomena. Restoring BR balance must start with understanding of the physiology behind the seven phases of BR during the day, starting in the morning and continuing to bedtime. At each phase, specific steps need to be taken in terms of personalized supplementation, diet, and lifestyle modulations tailoring to each body's specific clinical neurotransmitter volume, hormonal balance, receptor function, toxic load, body sensitivity, and assimilation capacity at that point in time to rebalance proper BR. The goal is to restore neurotransmitter balance to a state appropriate to the specific phase for the time of day to mimic the natural cycle as closely as possible.

Because most are already physically weak at this time from long standing insomnia, any rebalancing has to progress slowly. This is especially true in the beginning. Those who are in advanced stages of AFS are particularly vulnerable. Paradoxical or exaggerated reactions are common and have to be avoided. Expert close guidance and monitoring is required. Immediate adjustments are made in real time if possible. The rebalancing process usually only takes a few months in experienced hands.

Recovery tips through the Seven Daily Temporal BR Phases

Awakening Rhythm from 6 to 9 a.m.: Some people wake up refreshed in the morning having had a good night's sleep. Others wake up still tired, but begin to perk up after having breakfast and beginning their morning routine. Still others wake up refreshed, but drag through this phase. Regardless of where you fall, the body can start its BR rebalancing effort in this phase.

Increase energy using macro and micronutrition principles. Have a good breakfast when you wake up and start your day's activities. NT balance needs to be in an excitatory bias to get your body moving. The BR should be clear of yesterday's burdens from the overnight rest. The body is fresh as we start the new day. Start with some Adrenal Circulation and Adrenal Restorative Exercises to help the BR. Nutritional supplementation with the right compounds is key to helping the restorative process progress initially.

Recommendations for more energy in the morning:

- Vitamin B6

- Vitamin C

- DHEA

- Glutathione

- Glycine

- Pregnenolone

- Amino acid such as arginine

- Trace minerals

- Iodine

- Tyrosine

- Vitamin B5 and pantethine

- Vitamin D

- Thyroid glandular

- Adrenal cortex

- Zinc

- Selenium

- Vitamin B12

Morning Rhythm from 9 a.m. to noon: Your goal is to sustain your energy throughout the morning until lunch, while avoiding both anxiety and fatigue, which can occur in late morning as energy starts to wane and symptoms of hypoglycemia may appear. The overall neurotransmitter balance should become neutral as the awakening phase wears itself out.

Recommendations are to support your bodily functions as you continue awakening. As the morning progresses, enjoy a relaxing cup of warm broth or a light nutritious snack during this phase to prevent any BR disruption from metabolic imbalance. Supporting the spleen at this time is important, so you should have lentils or yams seasoned with cinnamon. Adrenal Yoga Exercise is recommended during this time. Adrenal Breathing Exercise is particularly important in midmorning to tone down any excessive NT excitation carryover from the awakening phase, such as from taking in coffee, glandulars, and stimulatory herbs like ashwagandha, rhodiola, maca, and ginseng.

Anxiety has a tendency to surface in late morning. Any liver or extracellular matrix congestion can make matters worse. Supplement considerations should focus on neutralizing any excitatory NT tone as well as relieving liver and extracellular matrix burden. Combat this and stabilize your neurotransmitters with these:

- GABA

- Magnesium

- Theanine

- 5-HTP

- Activated charcoal

- Clay

- High resistance water

- Fermented milk thistle

- Fish oil

- NAC

- Lipoic acid

Lunch Rhythm from noon to 2 p.m.: Make sure that you have a good lunch with enough calories to sustain you through the entire afternoon. The food choice should be biased towards more protein and fat and less carbohydrate. Salads with chicken, for example, are excellent choices for lunch. You should also supplement with the proper micronutrients, focusing on supporting continuous energy and preventing an imbalance in metabolism, which can bring on a food coma that occurs soon after lunch and disrupts the BR. Your NT balance should continue to be neutral and allow the nutrients from lunch to give you enough energy without depending on excitatory neurotransmitters to start the afternoon activities.

Recommendations for this phase: It would be best to enjoy a nice relaxing lunch and take a twenty-minute power nap immediately thereafter. The heart doesn't respond well to emotional or physical heat during this phase so you need to avoid:

- Caffeine

- Stress

- Intense exercise

- Anything that raises blood pressure

Afternoon Rhythm from 2 to 5 p.m.: You need to support your energy flow in mid-afternoon and try to prevent any slumps in energy that could set off an alarm response causing an excessive release of norepinephrine and epinephrine and trigger an adrenal crash. Have an afternoon snack that includes complex carbohydrates. Take a twenty to thirty minute afternoon nap around 3 p.m. The NT balance should be a bit excitatory to make sure your body has enough reserve energy to sustain you throughout the afternoon if it's not possible to take a nap. The net BR balance is maintained on a cruising mode.

Recommendations for sustaining you throughout the afternoon: It's important to have a strong bladder during this time (for storing and secreting urine). The bladder is nourished with salty foods so have a bowl of soup with a lot of liquid broth like miso or vegetable. This will keep the bladder and the kidneys (the paired organs) strong.

To combat an afternoon slump in energy and avoid metabolic imbalance:

- Arginine

- Chromium

- Glutamine

- Holy basil

- Hydrolyzed collagen type 1 and 3

- Milk thistle

- Minerals such as marine phytoplankton

- Amino acid such as arginine and glutamine

- DHEA

- Pregnenolone

- Magnesium and theanine for anxiety carryover

Dinner Rhythm from 6 to 9 p.m.: The objective here is to gradually reduce your excitatory NT tone through dinnertime.

Ensure the smooth assimilation of food without any metabolic dysregulation, which can trigger internal inflammation. Your overall NT balance should be slightly inhibitory in order to maintain a neutral BR, setting the stage for slowdown at the end of the day.

Recommendations for relaxing and easing into a sleep mode: You may take some time for meditation, reading, light stretching or cuddling.

To combat early evening anxiety:

- 5-HTP

- Fish oil

- GABA in a low dose

- Magnesium

- Taurine

- Theanine

- Chromium

Those suffering from high cortisol at night should commence cortisol lowering with natural compounds that have a lagging effect such as phosphatidylserine as well as continue Adrenal Breathing Exercises.

Sleep Onset Rhythm from 9 p.m. to 2 a.m.: This is the time for the body to unwind. Your NTs should be moving towards a more inhibitory tone with acetylcholine acting as the main NT needed for the parasympathetic nervous system to maintain the proper state for digestion and rest.

Take a small snack rich in protein and fat right before sleep. Almond milk and nuts are excellent choices. This will help stabilize blood sugar and prevent metabolic imbalances that can occur a few hours later.

Recommendations to combat sleep onset insomnia (SOI):

- 5-HTP

- Arginine

- Fish oil

- GABA in small to moderate doses

- Magnesium

- Niacin

- Passion flower

- Phosphatidylserine

- Melatonin

- Progesterone

- Fermented herbs such as valerian root

- Vitamin D may be helpful for those with history of paradoxical reactions.

- Those with low cortisol can consider licorice and grapefruit juice.

Those with high cortisol can consider phosphatidylserine (PS) and bioactive milk peptides. Bioactive milk peptides can be taken at bedtime, but PS should be taken a few hours before as well as at bedtime.

Sleep Maintenance Rhythm from 2 to 6 a.m.: At this time, the body requires an ample supply of the needed inhibitory NTs, which combat any residual excitatory stimuli that may cause wakefulness during the night. We want to prevent the BR from receiving any stimulation. Metabolic imbalances can cause frequent awakenings and your bedtime snack should be helpful in preventing this from triggering sleeplessness during this period.

Recommendations to combat sleep maintenance insomnia (SMI):

- 5-HTP (time-release form)
- Chromium polynicotinate (time-release form)
- Melatonin (time-release form)
- Glycine in high doses to saturate the body can be considered and taken at this time to support sleep for those with sleep maintenance insomnia
- Magnesium
- Niacinamide
- Passion flower
- Taurine
- Glycine
- Inositol
- Fish oil
- Bioactive milk peptides

Proper timing of taking sleep aids is important. Glycine, for example, should be taken at bedtime and not at the time of awakening in the middle of the night because of a lagging effect. We can also take advantage of time release forms of melatonin and 5-HTP so their onset of action can be timed a few hours after going to sleep.

This phase is the most challenging because frequent awakenings and the inability to return to sleep is a sure recipe for fatigue the next day. Higher and frequent doses of supplementation and snacks throughout the night may be required. The Adrenal Breathing Exercise is very valuable at this time.

Five Reasons why Self-Directed Programs Fail

Proper BR balance, especially in cases of severe insomnia, requires a comprehensive plan addressing the needs of each of the seven temporal BR phases of the day. This is done in order to maintain an overall daily rhythm that is natural, stable and consistent. This comprehensive plan requires extensive clinical experience. Even in the best of hands, some trial and error is required due to the lack of accurate laboratory tests for guidance in addition to each body's unique setting.

Many have tried self-navigating through a variety of natural compounds but failed to restore BR properly. Here are five common reasons for failure:

- First, most are not versed in understanding the specific physiological pathway of each nutrient, resulting in the wrong choice. For example, taurine has NT inhibitory effects, but it is also a natural diuretic and increases excretion of water from the body. Taking it at nighttime may help sleep, however, it can also lead to increased awakenings due to the need for frequent urination. Another example is 5-HTP. It tends to work better in the evening while GABA is better during the day. Proper selection of nutrients timed specifically for each phase will greatly enhance success.

- Second, the approach of using targeted single nutrients works only in the mildest of cases. For example, melatonin alone may work well in early stages of AFS when BR disruption is mild. In a setting of advanced AFS, insomnia is already well entrenched. Many have already been put on sleep medications by their physicians after sleep aids fail. Different nutritional cocktails specific for the needs of each of the seven temporal BR phases of the day are usually required in order to reset the BR properly, especially in the beginning.

- Third, dosage requirements vary greatly from person to person. Melatonin at 3 mg may work well for one person but is completely inadequate for another who may do much better at a lower dose of say, 0.3 mg, or a higher dose of 30 mg. In other words, some compounds, like melatonin, are not linear in their dose response curve. More is not necessarily better.

- Fourth, certain compounds are more effective when taken by various delivery methods. For example, sublingual melatonin is more effective, especially in high doses, than capsules or pills because they contain less inert substances called binders and fillers required during the manufacturing process. Excessive binders and fillers can trigger vivid dreams and nightmares in those who have a sensitive pineal gland.

- Finally, proper timing is required to maximize the effectiveness of each natural compound. For example, the phosphorylated form of phosphatidylserine (PS) is more effective to lower cortisol at night as compared to the non-phosphorylated form. However, there is a four to six hour lag period from time of intake to bio activation. As such, it should be taken well before bedtime to be most effective.

In addition to the above five parameters, there is danger in blind supplementation without consideration for several important additional factors regarding the constitution: stage of AFS, receptor site response, GI assimilation state, sleep medication dependency, extracellular matrix pollution and liver burden. Failures to consider these factors are common clinical mistakes resulting in improper doses and clinical failure.

A successful comprehensive BR rebalancing program is highly intricate and requires extensive clinical experience in both BR and AFS. Because dosage varies so widely from person to person, a detailed clinical history is key to assessing the right starting dose and combination of compounds. Most self-directed programs fail, not because of the lack of tools but due to operator inexperience, resulting in a worsening outcome over time. Conversely, we are happy to report that most cases of BR and severe insomnia can be improved with natural compounds when recovery is properly structured and executed.

Key Points to Remember:

Chronobiology is the study of biological rhythms (BR) that govern the speed and frequency of many biological processes. Among the most important is the daily circadian rhythm.

Any disruption of homeostasis can disrupt the body's BR. The most common sign of BR disruption is insomnia. BR disruption can further effect negative changes in metabolism, mood and energy.

There are seven distinct modes of operation in our daily BR: awakening, morning, lunch, afternoon, dinner, sleep onset and sleep maintenance.

Proper restoration of BR, if it is disrupted, requires attending to each of these seven stages by nudging neurotransmitter balance towards the correct state for each of these rhythms. This can be achieved by using a cocktail of complementary nutrients customized to each body and specific state. Similar to MTHFR, pyroluria is another laboratory based assessment alternative practitioners explore when AFS sufferers are reaching for any possible answers.

Defining Our Terms

Throughout Adrenal Fatigue Syndrome, you will come upon certain terms and words that might or might not be familiar to you. Some terms come up in the text frequently, while others appear only once or twice. Rather than include a glossary at the end of the book, we decided to use this chapter to offer some easy, working definitions of commonly used terms. That way you can refresh your memory as they appear within the book. For example, throughout the text we refer to the components of the body's nervous system, and the definitions below will serve as a convenient reference. In other cases, we've defined terms we didn't define thoroughly when first seen in the text because they were used less often and we didn't want to stop the flow of information. Therefore, we added them to the list below. We also combined definitions of terms that logically fit together, rather than maintaining a strict glossary-style alphabetical order.

Acute/Chronic: When symptoms appear suddenly, we consider it an acute condition. For example, some common infections, such as colds, influenza, and pneumonia, come on quickly. The symptoms run their course and disappear as the body heals. Anaphylaxis shock is an acute allergic reaction to an allergen, and may be a life-threatening episode in an allergy considered to be chronic, that is, an ongoing condition. Many conditions have both acute and chronic components.

Diabetes is a chronic condition with long term implications, but acute episodes of blood sugar/insulin dysregulation can bring on symptoms, such as fainting or severe weakness, serious enough to require emergency room visits. Rheumatoid arthritis and cardiovascular disease have both acute and chronic components. Avoiding acute episodes is one goal of managing chronic diseases.

Adaptogen: The ability to modulate and adjust to conditions as they change, whether or not these conditions are optimal. In the context of herbs, the term usually refers to the ability to bring the biochemical function back to normal, no matter if it is too high or too low.

Anabolic/Catabolic: Anabolic is the buildup phase of metabolism, in that our tissues are synthesized from the proteins and other substances we provide. Catabolic is the breakdown phase of metabolism, in which the body supplies energy from the materials we have provided.

Autoimmune disorders: Many conditions, from rheumatoid arthritis to lupus to common allergies, result from the body's complex immune system. This system normally reacts to and works toward eradicating substances it perceives as "invaders." An autoimmune response occurs when the normal response is interrupted or disturbed and the immune system reacts to the body's tissues as invaders.

Challenge: Specific tests or protocols designed to prove or disprove a hypothesis.

Clearance: A measure of kidney and liver function. This refers to clearing a unit of a specific compound from a specific volume of plasma. The lower the clearance, the more compromised the function.

Crash: An abrupt state of reduced energy output and severe fatigue as the body reverts back to a simplistic form of function to conserve existing energy.

Decompensation: In medicine, when a previously working organ system or structure deteriorates, we call this decompensation. It can occur because of illness, stress, or aging. Compensating means the organ still tries to function despite the stressors. As Adrenal Fatigue Syndrome advances, the adrenals and other organ systems eventually begin to decompensate, potentially bringing on many confusing symptoms and organ system disorders.

Dysfunction: Impairment of a physiological function.

Dysregulation: Impairment of a physiological regulatory mechanism.

Metabolism: The overall term for the physical and chemical processes by which we produce, maintain, or breakdown the body's material substances.

Metabolites: The byproducts or results of metabolism. In addition, a metabolite is a product of metabolism that is more or less toxic to the organism producing it.

The Nervous System

The central nervous system (CNS): The portion of the nervous system that consists of the brain and spinal cord. The CNS gathers, stores, and controls information and is involved in all bodily and psychological functions, from breathing and walking to experiencing sadness and joy.

The peripheral nervous system: Consists of nerves and ganglia outside the CNS. It is divided into two parts: the somatic nervous system, which regulates musculoskeletal functions that help us deal with the outside world, and the autonomic nervous system (ANS), which regulates functions of the smooth muscles and glands within the body as described below.

Autonomic nervous system (ANS): The component of the nervous system that regulates involuntary actions, meaning we don't consciously control them, including heart and glandular activity. Multiple branches exist, the key ones being the sympathetic nervous system (SNS), the parasympathetic nervous system (PNS), and the adrenomedullary hormonal system (AHS).

Recovery cycle: When pertaining to Adrenal Fatigue Syndrome, recovery is the period immediately following a crash. Individuals will likely experience many cycles as they recover.

Stress: Put simply, stress is an individual's response to physical challenges, exertion, and events that create internal emotional pressure. We sometimes refer to the external events or circumstances as stressors, but our reactions are the source of stress, not the event itself.

Subclinical: Some conditions stay below the threshold at which we can detect and measure clinical signs and symptoms. For example, diabetes, hypertension, and hypothyroidism often produce symptoms, but clinical tests often show results in the normal range. We refer to this as a subclinical state. However, if left unattended, the condition can eventually worsen and abnormalities can appear on tests, hence, providing clinical evidence of their presence.

Unfortunately, subclinical states often occur but are ignored because the conditions are allowed to advance untreated until testing "proves" that the symptoms are real. In Adrenal Fatigue Syndrome, current testing techniques may produce results that look like there is normal adrenal function all the way up to adrenal failure. Therefore, we don't recommend relying on lab results as the final answer in diagnosing complex medical conditions and, in particular, AFS.

We hope these definitions will help you get the most from this book. Now, we begin discussing other issues related to AFS, as well as the stages of Adrenal Fatigue Syndrome.

The Stages of Adrenal Fatigue Syndrome: Overview

Without question, Adrenal Fatigue Syndrome, with its myriad manifestations, is both confusing and perplexing, a situation made worse by the lack of consistency in the way we refer to the condition. We use Adrenal Fatigue Syndrome as the overall name. Stages 3 and 4 refer to advanced AFS, and we call Stage 3 and its phases, Adrenal Exhaustion. Stage 4 is referred to as Adrenal Failure. To avoid confusion, except for providing the basic definitions, we use the term Adrenal Exhaustion only when referring to Stage 3.

Bear in mind that the stages and phases of AFS overlap greatly. The boundaries are indistinct. They are presented here to help us clinically get a feel for the broad perspective as it is very easy to be overwhelmed and miss the big picture. These definitions should not be used as tools for diagnosis.

Stage 1: Alarm Reaction

In this stage, which can last days, months, years, and even decades, the body periodically is alarmed by stressors and mounts an aggressive anti-stress response to reduce stress levels. (The stressors could be physical or psychological, or, typically, a combination of stressors that trigger the alarm reaction.) Common examples include events of daily life we often take for granted as normal, such as change of career, physical relocation, excessive exercise, and skipping meals on a regular basis. Some physicians refer to this as the "early fatigue" stage. In this state, brain norepinephrine output is increased, leading to a state of arousal and alertness. We use this alertness to keep us awake when it is time to go to sleep. We also see increased ACTH (a hormone produced by the anterior lobe of the pituitary gland), which stimulates the adrenal cortex into making more cortisol, DHEA, pregnenolone, and aldosterone, among others. These hormones' collective physiological actions result in a second wind to keep us going physically and emotionally when it is actually time to rest.

Individuals do not report symptoms at this stage, and their daily activities are unaffected, although they may note feeling tired. In order to maintain or boost their energy level, many rely on coffee or other caffeinated drinks to start their day. They may find they need increasing amounts of caffeine to feel revved up for the day. Unfortunately, the social acceptance of addiction to coffee gives us the excuse to carry a coffee cup around in the office. Some even consider this type of external stimulant normal. In fact, not to be part of the coffee culture can be considered unsociable.

Stage 1 is a common occurrence. Because the body's stress response is effective and no damage is perceived, no attention is paid to the fine detail of how the body is already drawing on its nutritional reserves at this stage. Almost all adults at one point or another have multiple such experiences. Many already have their first experience in their teenage years on retrospect. As long as the stress lessens and the normal rhythm of daily life returns, most people in this stage recover with extra rest. Most individuals pass in and out of Stage 1 without realizing they have experienced even a brief episode of adrenal fatigue. Routine blood laboratory tests are normal. Saliva cortisol testing is generally normal as well, but the morning cortisol usually starts trending up as Stage 1 progresses. In the absence of any outward symptoms other than occasional fatigue, this lack of energy is compensated by the socially acceptable use of stimuli to boost energy. Unfortunately, based on the premise that stimulating energy with coffee and sweets is harmless, for the most part, our society has inadvertently condoned this approach. In reality, suppressing symptoms only worsens the progression of those with Stage 1 AFS over time.

Stage 2: Resistance Response

Greater exposure to life stress, or psychological vulnerability to stress, increases cortisol demand. The neuroendocrine response is to put the HPA axis on overdrive to increase output of cortisol and other anti-stress hormones. Socioeconomic and psychosocial handicaps are probably central inducers of hyperactivity of the HPA axis. Alcohol, smoking, and traits of psychiatric disease may also be involved. The HPA axis starts to be overtaxed but at this stage is not yet dysfunctional.

Cortisol is the primary anti-stress hormone systemically. Its release from the adrenal glands helps to provide for and regulate our fuel requirement during stress. At the same time, it helps reduce inflammation and calm the nerves during highly stressful events. It serves as both an acceleration and braking mechanism at the same time via different pathways, ensuring our ability to successfully deal with stress and yet have normal physiological functioning. This is a temporary fix, however. One cannot drive a car successfully without damage over time if one foot is applied on the gas pedal, and the other one is applied on the brakes at the same time, though in varying degrees.

What makes this stage so dangerous is that much of the damage is subclinical and usually goes totally unnoticed. On the outside, one looks perfectly fine, but internal cellular damage is well under way.

Stage 2 often starts in the twenties or thirties and usually lasts for years into decades. Since, like Stage 1, it often goes undetected, it most often is evident only in retrospect. Intermittent fatigue, borderline or abnormal lipid panels, normal to borderline high blood pressure symptoms, and weight gain suggestive of reduced metabolism are treated as separate isolated problems, often with medications. The AFS picture is usually missed, especially early on. Most in this stage continue with their normal and active life on this track, thinking that all is well. Without considering AFS, they may be continually and unknowingly driving themselves into a path of slow destruction as cellular damage advances.

Many in lifelong Stage 2 are unaware of the internal dysfunction caused by stress, but as aging sets in, borderline signs and symptoms may become more prevalent. By midlife, many are physically showing gross signs of central obesity with a "muffin top" belly or "spare tire" in the abdominal area, accompanied by lack of vitality and tolerance for exercise, hyperlipidemia (high cholesterol), dysglycemia (abnormal glucose level), mild but worsening food sensitivities, mild insomnia, and inability to lose weight despite strenuous exercise.

It is important to remember that the absence of fatigue as the predominant symptom in Stage 2 does not mean that the body is not under stress. The body's well equipped neuroendocrine compensatory response is simply working extra hard and has successfully overcome stressors. This results in a relatively normal state of energy flow. Therefore, most at this stage are mislead into thinking that all is well.

Stage 3: Adrenal Exhaustion

Recall in Stage 2 that unrelenting stress increases cortisol output from the adrenal glands. After peaking, the cortisol level starts to drop. Despite rising ACTH production from the pituitary gland and ongoing HPA axis stimulation, the adrenals are no longer able to keep up with the body's increased demand for cortisol production. Moderate to severe persistent fatigue is the norm as the body enters Stage 3, Adrenal Exhaustion. This stage is also called Neuroendocrine Exhaustion as the neuroendocrine system is now on full throttle, with eventual breakdown as this stage progresses. This stage may develop over a period of years as well, which is why lifestyle issues are so important in analyzing and discussing AFS.

As stage 3 progresses, total cortisol output drops below normal, and DHEA falls far below average. A twenty-four hour saliva cortisol test is likely to show a cortisol curve that has a tendency to flatten as AFS advances. In addition to the morning cortisol level being low, the nighttime cortisol level is usually reduced as well. The body's nervous and endocrine systems progressively become more dysregulated as this stage advances. The HPA axis becomes dysfunctional and eventually burns out.

The 4 Phases of Stage 3

In Stage 3A, mild fatigue is constant, and the person could have low thyroid, or a woman could experience premenstrual syndrome (PMS). Rest usually doesn't bring about total recovery, but individuals in this stage function at about 75-100 percent of normal capacity.

In Stage 3B, mild to moderate fatigue is constant and these individuals do not get 100 percent recovery with rest. In terms of daily activities, they function at about 50-75 percent capacity. Symptoms of thyroid problems, estrogen dominance, and low libido often occur concurrently. Exercise becomes problematic.

In Stage 3C, the capacity to carry out normal activities is severely curtailed, down to 25-50 percent. These individuals might have to work part time, or often they are unable to work, or they try to work from home. By late Stage 3C, the ANS may itself be dysfunction due to overwork. Along with previous hormonal axes imbalances and receptor site dysregulation, the body is left with impaired metabolic, clearance, and detoxification pathways. This damage often gives rise to paradoxical, unpredictable, and exaggerated reactions and out- comes. For example, a person might have reactive blood sugar imbalances, that is, a quick rise in blood sugar after a meal, followed by a precipitous drop. Blood pressure might become fragile and unstable. It might drop suddenly when going from a supine to a sitting position (postural hypotension) along with a rapid increase in the heart rate, a phenomenon resembling subclinical POTS (postural orthostatic tachycardia syndrome).

Symptoms indicative of advanced Adrenal Exhaustion that is associated with subclinical metabolic derangement such as heart palpitations, dizziness, sudden onset of anxiety, a feeling of being wired-and-tired, internal dysbiosis (imbalance in intestinal flora), acid-based imbalances, and adrenaline rushes. We may also see fluid and electrolyte imbalance, such as insufficient sodium (salt) in fluids outside the cells (hyponatremia).

In Stage 3D, most are unable to work and are incapacitated. The body's key hormones, such as cortisol and aldosterone, might fall close or below the minimum required reserve for normal function and output. When this occurs, the body may down-regulate the amount of hormones needed in order to preserve what is on hand for only the most essential body functions. Extreme fatigue is common. We characterize this near failure state as Stage 3D. The body goes into full surrender as it gives up trying and simply does what it can to reduce energy-out to stay alive. In other words, the body is now in survival mode.

At 3D many sufferers are essentially bedridden. Those with symptoms of Stage3D are in an extremely sensitive state, often feeling worse if they take supplements, for example. In addition, they often are in a catabolic state, which means the body's protein is breaking down and these individuals are losing weight. Digestion is usually breaking down, too, and these people may become constipated or unable to tolerate regular food well.

Stage 4: Adrenal Failure

Eventually, the adrenals and the neuroendocrine system become totally worn out and are defeated in their attempt to overcome stress. Metabolic pathway damage and toxic metabolite built up becomes unrelenting. The body surrenders as the only viable option for survival. This stage is also called Neuroendocrine Failure. When Adrenal Fatigue Syndrome has advanced to this stage, the line between AFS and subclinical and clinical Addison's disease, also called adrenal insufficiency, can be blurry. We may see the emergence of typical symptoms of Addison's disease: extreme fatigue, weight loss, muscle weakness, loss of appetite, nausea, vomiting, hypoglycemia, headache, sweating, irregular menstrual cycles, depression, orthostatic hypotension, dehydration, and electrolyte imbalances. The body appears to have lost its normal homeostasis and is breaking down. Intensive conventional multi-disciplinary medical attention is needed to achieve stabilization well beyond what can be done naturally. Hospitalization may be required. This stage will not be our concern in Adrenal Fatigue Syndrome.

3-Minute Adrenal Fatigue Test

Here is a checklist of common symptoms associated with Adrenal Fatigue Syndrome. Check the boxes that are applicable and record your score below, Learn what it means for your health personally and what you may need to do if there are signs of suffering from Adrenal Fatigue Syndrome.

☐ Tendency to gain weight especially at the waist and in-ability to lose it.

☐ High frequency of getting the flu and other respiratory diseases that tend to last longer than usual.

☐ Reduced sex drive.

☐ Lightheaded when rising from a supine position.

☐ Unable to remember things and unclear thinking.

☐ Lack of energy in the mornings and also in the afternoon between 3 and 5:00 PM.

☐ Feel better suddenly for a brief period after a meal.

☐ Need coffee or stimulants to get going in the morning.

☐ Craving for salty, fatty, and high protein food such as meat and cheese.

☐ Increased symptoms of PMS for women; periods are heavy and then stop, or almost stop on the 4th day, only to start to flow again on the 5th or 6th day.

☐ Pain in the upper back or neck for no apparent reasons. Easily startled.

☐ Decreased ability to handle stress and responsibilities.

Body temperature is off balance; hands and feet feel cold, face feels warm, or hot flashes.

☐ Unexplained hair loss.

☐ Tendency to tremble when under pressure. Multiple allergies such as asthma, hay fever, skin rashes, eczema, hives, and food sensitivity.

Enter the number of checkmarks you have made: _____

What Does Your Score Mean?

If your score is 4 or below, chances are you do not have Adrenal Fatigue Syndrome unless your symptoms are quite severe. There may be other dysfunction in place. Adrenal Fatigue Syndrome is unlikely to be significantly involved, although we can't be sure without a detailed history. You can adopt many of the dietary and lifestyle recommendations in our book Adrenal Fatigue Syndrome or various articles we have online at DrLam. com. Most supplements are generally well tolerated if your doctor approves. If you do not improve within a reasonable amount of time, write to us through our website with your score and what you did. We will give you our thoughts in confidence.

If your score is 5-9, you may or may not have Adrenal Fatigue Syndrome. Many conditions mimic AFS, so if you have not already done so, visit your doctor for further medical investigation. If you are given a clean bill of health but remain symptomatic, consider Adrenal Fatigue Syndrome. The higher your score on the test, the higher your risk of Adrenal Fatigue Syndrome. You also can adopt many of the dietary and lifestyle recommendations mentioned in our book Adrenal Fatigue Syndrome, but be cautious when it comes to nutritional supplementation, as they can worsen the condition if not properly used. If you are not sure where you stand or what to do, then write directly and privately to us online through our website (DrLam.com) with your score and a brief history. We'll give you our assessment and suggestions in confidence.

If your score is 10 or above, it is imperative that you become fully educated about Adrenal Fatigue Syndrome and alert your doctor about this condition. The more severe your symptoms, the more dysfunctional your adrenal glands likely are. We do not recommend self-navigation as it often makes the condition worse over time. If you cannot find someone knowledgeable to help you, if you fail to improve on your recovery plan, and are not sure where you stand or what to do next, then write to us directly and privately through our website (www.DrLam.com). Let us know your score, a detailed medical history, and your main complaints. We will reply to you in confidence and give you some guidance.

This free test is also available online at our website: www.DrLam.com/adrenal-fatigue-test.asp.

Suggested Reading and Resources

I n addition to the books, CDs and DVDs listed in the front of Adrenal Fatigue Syndrome, here are additional free readings and resources from our website, www.DrLam.com/afs/. When on the site, just click on the topic of interest. Each will help you understand the scientific basis of our approach to Adrenal Fatigue Syndrome we take throughout this book.

- Acidosis Aging Brain Andropause

- Atrial Fibrillation

- Beef, Chicken, or Fish

- Blood Thinners and Nutritional Supplements

- Chelation Cholesterol Dehydration Detoxification DHEA Diabetes

- Eggs — Good for your body?

- Endometriosis

- Nutritional Supplements — To Take or Not?

- Omega 3 Fatty Acid Oral Health Progesterone

- The Big Fat Lie

- Estrogen Dominance

- Fibroids

- Heart Disease Prevention — A Complete Nutritional Approach

- Hypothyroidism Insulin and Aging: Magnesium and

Aging

- Menopause
- Metabolic Syndrome
- Milk — The Perfect Food?
- My Doctor Is Killing Me
- New Markers of Cardiovascular Disease
- Nutritional Medicine
- Upper Limits Vitamin C and E Intake
- Water
- Where to Buy Supplements
- Why Conventional Medicine Rejects Adrenal Fatigue Syndrome

After Recovery

After your recovery from Adrenal Fatigue Syndrome, the natural progression is to embark on an anti-aging program where you begin to reverse the biological clock naturally, while keeping AFS at bay. We have a complete library on this in our website. The following articles are helpful and found also on www.DrLam.com/afs/.

Anti-aging Program

- Dr. Lam's Smoothie Recipe Anti-aging Strategies
- Customized Exercise Routine
- Blood Type Diet
- Links to Various Health Centers Osteoporosis

- Calories That Count
- Woman's Optimal Daily Allowance
- Men's Optimal Daily Allowance
- Links to Natural Protocols for Common Health Conditions

For the Avid Reader in Natural Health

You can download our free online ebooks from our home page at www.DrLam.com:

- *Beating Cancer with Natural Medicine*
- *5 Proven Secrets to Longevity*

Other Useful Links

New information and links on natural health and Adrenal Fatigue Syndrome are regularly added to our website library. These include many nonprofit educational organizations, links to scientific journals, periodicals, and additional recommended books. Here is the link: www.DrLam.com/links.asp

Chapter Notes

Chapter 1

Agranoff, Bernard W. (22 July 2003). "History of Neurochemistry." Encyclopedia of Life Sciences.

Antunes-Rodrigues, José; Castro, Margaret De; Elias, Lucila L. K.; Valença, Marcelo M.; McCann, Samuel M. (1 January 2004). "Neuroendocrine Control of Body Fluid Metabolism."

"Epigenetics and the Human Brain." Genetics Science and Learning Center at The University of Utah. Retrieved 10 November 2013.

Ratka, Anna; Sutanto, Winardi; Bloemers, Margreet; de Kloet, Ronald, (1989). "On the Role of Brain Mineralocorticoid (Type I) and Glucocorticoid (Type II) Receptors in Neuroendocrine Regulation."

Siegel, George J.; Albers, R.W.; Brady, S.T.; Price, D.L., (2006). Basic Neurochemistry, 7th Ed. Academic Press.

Chapter 2

Bischoff, S.C., Dahinden, C.A. "C-kit ligand: A unique potentiator of mediator release by human lung mast cells." J Exp Med. 175 (1992):237

Caraceni, A., Grassi, L. Delirium: Acute Confusional States in Palliative Medicine. (Oxford: Oxford University Press; 2011):11

Costa, J.J., Demetri, G.D., Harrist, T.J., et al. "Recombinant human stem cell factor (kit ligand) promotes human mast cell and melanocyte hyperplasia and functional activation in vivo." J Exp Med 183 (1996):2681

Fleminger, S. "Remembering delirium." The British Journal of Psychiatry. 180(1) (2002):4-5

Fogarty, J.E. A Barefoot Doctor's Manual: The American Translation of the Official Chinese Paramedical Manual. (Philadelphia: Running Press; 1990)

Lishman, W.A., Organic Psychiatry: The Psychological Consequences of Cerebral Disorder. (Hoboken: John Wiley & Sons; 1998):4

Neufeld, W.P. The Liver Causes Heart Attack. (Surrey: Morning Dawn Publishing; 1987)

Posner, J.B., Clifford B.S., Schiff, N., Plum, F. Plum and Posner's Diagnosis of Stupor and Coma (4th edition). (Oxford: Oxford University Press; 2007):8

Sedman, G. "Theories of Depersonalization: A Re-appraisal." The British Journal of Psychiatry 117(536) (2970):1-14

Selkurt, E.E. Physiology, 2nd edition. (Boston: Little, Brown and Company; 1966)

Yudofsky, S.C., Hales, R.E. The American Psychiatric Publishing textbook of neuropsychiatry and behavioral neurosciences. (Washington, DC: American Psychiatric Pub.; 2008):449

Chapter 3

Andrews, J. International Symposium on Nitric Oxide (Toronto: MaRS Discovery District; May 27-28, 2010)

Fleet, R.P., Dupuis, G., Marchand, A., Burelle, D., Beitman, B.D. "Panic disorder, chest pain and coronary artery disease: literature review." Can J Cardiol. 10(8) (1994):827

Goddard, A.W., Mason, G.F., Appel, M., et al. "Impaired GABA neuronal response to acute benzodiazepine administration in panic disorder." Am J Psychiatry. 161 (2004):2186

Gross, L. ""Supporting" Players Take the Lead in Protecting the Overstimulated Brain." PLoS Biology. 4(11) (2006)

Katon, W., Ries, R.K., Kleinman, A. "The prevalence of somatization in primary care." Compr Psychiatry. 25 (1984):208

Kolb, B., Whishaw, I.Q. An introduction to brain and behavior (4th edition). (New York: Worth Publishers; 2014):150-151

Roy-Byrne, P.P., Cowley, D.S. "Course and outcome in panic disorder: a review of recent follow-up studies." Anxiety 1 (1994-1995):151

Sherbourne, C.D., Sullivan, G., Craske, M.G., et al. "Functioning and disability levels in primary care out-patients with one or more anxiety disorders." Psychol Med. 11 (2010):1

Sherbourne, C.D., Wells, K.B., Judd, L.L. "Functioning and well-being of patients with panic disorder." Am J Psychiatry. 153 (1996):213

Sheehan, D.V. "Current concepts in psychiatry. Panic attacks and phobias." N Engl J Med. 307 (1982):156

Smoller, J.W., Pollack, M.H., Wassertheil-Smoller, S., et al. "Panic attacks and risk of incident cardiovascular events among postmenopausal women in the Women's Health Initiative Observational Study." Arch Gen Psychiatry. 64 (2007):1153

Watt, M.C., Stewart, S.H., Cox, B.J. "A retrospective study of the learning history origins of anxiety sensitivity." Behav Res Ther. 36 (1998):505

Chapter 4

Alvaro, P.K., Roberts, R.M., Harris, J.K. "A Systematic Review Assessing Bidirectionality between Sleep Disturbances, Anxiety and Depression." Sleep. 36 (2013):1059

Bonnet, M.H., Arand, D.K. "Heart rate variability in insomniacs and matched normal sleepers." Psychosom Med. 60 (1998):610

Brower, K.J., Aldrich, M.S., Robinson, E.A., et al. "Insomnia, self-medication, and relapse to alcoholism." Am J Psychiatry. 158 (2001):399

Costa e Silva, J.A., Chase, M., Sartorius, N., Roth, T. "Special report from a symposium held by the World Health Organization and the World Federation of Sleep Research Societies: an overview of insomnias and related disorders-recognition, epidemiology, and rational management." Sleep 19 (1996):412

Fava, M., McCall, W.V., Krystal, A., et al. "The natural history of insomnia: a population-based 3-year longitudinal study." Arch Intern Med 169 (2009):447

Ford, D.E., Kamerow, D.B. "Epidemiologic study of sleep disturbances and psychiatric disorders. An opportunity for prevention?" JAMA 262 (1989):1479

Krystal, A.D. "Psychiatric comorbidity: the case for treating insomnia." Sleep Med Clin 1 (2006):359

Parthasarathy, S., Vasquez, M.M., Halonen, M., et al. "Persistent insomnia is associated with mortality risk." Am J Med 128 (2015):268

Roehrs, T., Papineau, K., Rosenthal, L., Roth, T. "Ethanol as a hypnotic in insomniacs: self administration and effects on sleep and mood." Neuropsychopharmacology. 20 (1999):279

Sateia, M.J. "International classification of sleep disorders-Third Edition: highlights and modifications." Chest 146 (2014):1387

About the Authors

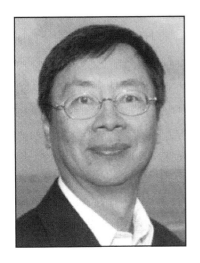

Michael Lam, MD, MPH, ABAAM, is a western trained physician specializing in nutritional and anti-aging medicine. Dr. Lam received his Bachelor of Science degree from Oregon State University, and his Doctor of Medicine degree from the Loma Linda University School of Medicine in California. He also holds a Master's degree in Public Health. He is board certified by the American Board of Anti-Aging Medicine where he has also served as a board examiner. Dr. Lam is a pioneer in using nontoxic, natural compounds to promote the healing of many age-related degenerative conditions. He utilizes optimum blends of nutritional supplementation that manipulate food, vitamins, natural hormones, herbs, enzymes, and minerals into specific protocols to rejuvenate cellular function. Dr. Lam was first to coin the term, ovarian-adrenal-thyroid (OAT) hormone axis, and to describe its imbalances. He was first to scientifically tie in Adrenal Fatigue Syndrome (AFS) as part of the overall neuroendocrine stress response continuum of the body. He systematized the clinical significance and coined the various phases of Adrenal Exhaustion. He has written 6 books, including Adrenal Fatigue Syndrome: Reclaim Your Energy and Vitality with Clinically Proven Natural Programs, Central Nervous System Disruptions of Adrenal Fatigue Syndrome, The Five Proven Secrets to Longevity, Beating Cancer with Natural Medicine, How to Stay Young and Live Longer, and Estrogen Dominance. In 2001, Dr. Lam established www.

DrLam.com as a free, educational website on evidence-based alternative medicine for the public and for health professionals. It featured the world's most comprehensive library on AFS. Provided free as a public service, he has answered countless questions through the website on alternative health and AFS. His personal, telephone-based nutritional coaching services have enabled many around the world to regain control of their health using natural therapies.

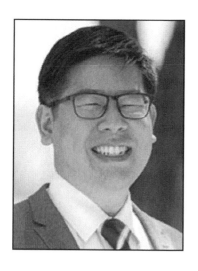

Dr. Justin Lam, ABAAHP, FMNM is a metabolic nutritionist specializing in Adrenal Fatigue. He earned his Bachelor of Science degree in Biology from Pacific Union College, California and his Doctor of Medicine degree from Ross University School of Medicine, a fully U.S. accredited medical school in Dominica. He is a diplomate in Anti-aging Medicine and board certified by the American Board of Anti-Aging Health Practitioners. He has completed a fellowship in Metabolic and Nutritional Medicine from the American Academy of Anti-Aging Medicine in educational partnership with George Washington University. He is a lifestyle health coach certified by the Metabolic Medical Institute. He is the son of Michael Lam, MD, recognized pioneer in adrenal fatigue, and is an integral part of Dr. Lam's worldwide telephone-based nutritional coaching team. His research focuses on the neuroendometabolic ramifications of exertion intolerance.

Dr. Lam's Adrenal Recovery Series

Dr. Lam has created a Mini-series of books as well as Singles for your use to aid in your recovery. Adrenal Fatigue Syndrome is a comprehensive guidebook. The Mini and Singles series allows you to have "select" sections that support and enhance your education and recovery. They are easier to carry with you for reference, allowing you to bookmark specific sections during your recovery program.

The Mini Series of paperback and e-books include:

- *Psychology of Adrenal Fatigue Syndrome: How the Mind-Body Connection Affects Your Recovery*

- *Anatomy of Adrenal Fatigue Syndrome: Clinical Stages 1 – 4*

- *Natural Therapeutics to Adrenal Fatigue Syndrome: Proper Use of Vitamins, Glandulars, Herbs, and Hormones*

- *Dietary and Lifestyle Therapeutics to Adrenal Fatigue Syndrome: Your Personal Recovery Toolbox*

- *Central Nervous System Disruptions of Adrenal Fatigue Syndrome*

- *Advanced Symptoms of Adrenal Fatigue Syndrome: A Metabolic Perspective*

- *Estrogen Dominance: Hormonal Imbalance of the 21st Century (Expanded Version)*

The Singles Series of e-books include:

- *Neuroendocrine Basis of Adrenal Fatigue Syndrome: The Physiology of Fatigue*

- *Adrenal Crashes: How to Prevent and Recover Quickly*

- *Diagnostic Testing for Adrenal Fatigue Syndrome: Everything You Need to Know*

- *Adrenal Fatigue Syndrome Progression and Case Study: What is Coming Ahead*

- *Your Constitution and Adrenal Fatigue Syndrome: How Your Genetic Makeup Can Affect Your Recovery*

- *Travel Tips and Adrenal Fatigue Syndrome: How to Avoid Adrenal Crashes*

- *Ovarian-Adrenal-Thyroid Axis Imbalance: Why Your Thyroid Medications May Not Be Working*

- *7 Adrenal Recovery Mistakes: What Successful Recovery Avoids*

- *Anti-aging and Adrenal Fatigue Syndrome:*

- *Incorporating an Anti-aging Program Into Your Recovery*

- *Myths of Adrenal Fatigue Syndrome: Separating the Facts from the Fiction*

Individual copies can be ordered fromDrLam.com as well as through online retailers.

Made in the
USA
Columbia, SC